Nancy Nix-Rice guides us to look good through photos, illustrations, and great copy. It's almost as if she's standing next to us, saying, "Try this!" No matter your age, style, and pocketbook, you'll find this your go-to fashion reference.

Nancy Zieman, Producer/Host of TV's *Sewing With Nancy* and founder of Nancy's Notions

Looking Good...Every Day takes *Looking Good* to another level. Nancy Nix-Rice's new approach through "points of connection" is unique and easy to understand, and hundreds of photos provide proof that this approach works. Filled with timeless principles of color, line, design, and proportion, *Looking Good...Every Day* helps women of all ages, shapes, and lifestyles make flattering choices while maximizing their wardrobe budget. This is a book every sewer and non-sewer alike should have!

Leslie Willmott
Image & Wardrobe Consultant,
Smart Women On The Go,
former corporate sales
executive, and co-author,
Clothes Sense

LOOKING GOOD
...every day

Style Solutions for
Real Women

My usual reaction to a new "style" book is to sit on my hands. After reading *Looking Good...Every Day*, I was ready to stand on a chair and yodel! Finally, a timeless reference book for women of all ages and sizes! This book, now, will be the text for my classes. Thank you, Nancy, for a job very well done.

Kathryn Brown CSI, *Sewing Instructor and Style Lecturer*

As a presentation skills trainer and coach, I work with women presenters to help them project confidence and credibility. Now I can't wait to recommend *Looking Good...Every Day* to them. This is such a powerful resource: It helps a woman evaluate what showcases her unique attributes. When she dresses and accessorizes to accentuate her best self, she'll discover that in the front of the room, the focus will be on her face and her communications, not on "OMG, what is she wearing?!" This book underscores that your presence is powerful when everything is connected—clothing, color, style, accessories. And I love how it shows you how to connect everything, step by colorfully illustrated step!

Barbara Busey, President, *Presentation Dynamics*

Looking Good...Every Day is a marvelous book that includes every topic you need to know for how to look great. Each chapter is detailed but easy to understand because of the superb quality of writing. The chapter on color showcases the importance of wearing a flattering color. This is a current and thorough textbook that should be in every image consultant's library.

Elaine Stoltz, AICI CIM

As an image consulting instructor who has used Nancy's original *Looking Good* book since 2000, I'm thrilled with this updated version. While reviewing the new copy, I got excited—the color pages really make a difference! The book is loaded with new information and the pictures throughout the book reflect a diverse group of women.... It is an easy and enjoyable book to read and the step-by-step guidelines with the body style will be an added bonus when I introduce students to body analysis.... I'm very pleased with the book and will look forward to when I can start using it for my image consulting class. The book is so comprehensive, I will continue to use it as an introduction to image consulting.

Kelly Armstrong, Image Consulting Instructor
Fashion Department, City College of San Francisco

This is a comprehensive, step-by-step volume for any woman who wants to know how to look her best, every day. Nancy Nix-Rice leads readers through the fundamental and essential style principles, from discovery to application to wardrobe maintenance. Readers learn to identify their innate assets and how to accentuate them no matter their lifestyle and budget. By using basic and timeless design concepts, readers (and wardrobe consultants) can make better selections for themselves, use their "ideal style connections" to choose the best from what's in fashion at the time, and thereby always Look Good, Every Day!

Dominique Isbecque, AICI, CIP,
Executive Director of Image Resource Center of NY LLC,
co-founder, Association of Image Consultants International (AICI)
Facilitator of the Certificate Program in Image Consulting at FIT
(Fashion Institute of Technology)

From the point of view of a fabric retailer, I found the sections relating to fabric choice, whether in ready-to-wear or custom sewing, filled with insightful and practical advice for consumers. Understanding fabrication, design and texture is essential to making good choices. In a world where we rely more and more on digital images to make our shopping selections, Nancy's discussion of scale, texture and print provides an indispensable guide to add to our decision-making toolbox.

Barb Blom, Owner, Sawyer Brook Distinctive Fabrics

Giving the reader the tools she needs to objectively assess her unique physical characteristics, *Looking Good...Every Day* offers every woman a step-by-step approach to discover her best colors, silhouettes and styles. Establishing points of connection further empowers her to draw conclusions based on the science of image rather than her own instinct, the makeover shows, or fashion magazines.

Carol Davidson, AICI CIP,
President & Chief Style Officer, StyleWorks of Union Square

A very useful and comprehensive guide for putting together—or refining—every aspect of your wardrobe from style to closets to shopping. Enough depth for the image "geeks," but accessible to all. The "Do's and Don'ts"—with illustrations—are particularly helpful. Food for study ... as well as for thought! A definite keeper.

Beryl Wing, AICI CIP,
Owner and Chief Strategy officer, The Image Authority

This book is like an encyclopedia—in the very best sense. It's packed full of information from A to Z for anyone trying to simplify the act of getting dressed. It's a great resource for garment sewers, but you don't have to be a sewer to use this book.

I love the modern approach that presents you with helpful apps and ways to use technology, if you choose, to make the process easier. And Nancy provides little exercises so you can easily analyze yourself and make all the connections you'll need to find those style solutions.

The illustrations and photos really make the book work because they so clearly show the points Nancy is making—like the amazing thing that can happen when you reposition a belt, tuck in a shirt, or add a little shoulder pad. It's well organized, too, so whether you read it from start to finish (which I recommend because Nancy has a great sense of humor and you'll enjoy the read) or just search out the sections on topics that trouble you the most, you can easily find what you're looking for.

If you've always wished for a friend to help you work through the process of learning to look the way you always knew you could, this book feels like that friend.

Mary Ray, Freelance Teacher, Writer, Designer
Contributing Editor, *Threads* magazine
Adjunct Instructor, Apparel Design & Merchandising,
Appalachian State University, Boone, NC

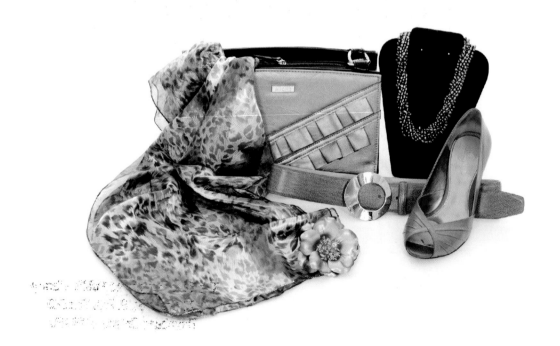

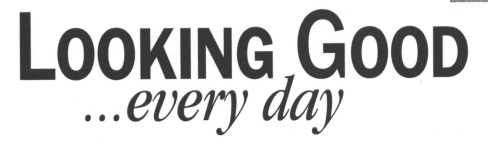

LOOKING GOOD
...every day

Style Solutions for Real Women

by Nancy Nix-Rice

Designed by Linda Wisner
Photography by Pati Palmer
Image Consulting and Styling by Ethel Harms
Illustration by Taylor Jean Engel and Kate Pryka
Editing by Pati Palmer
Copy Editing by Ann Gosch

Palmer/Pletsch PUBLISHING

This book would never exist without the collaboration of many talented individuals:

- Leslie Wood Willmott and Barbara Weiland Talbert, whose original volume, *Clothes Sense,* inspired this book.
- Publisher and book photographer, Pati Palmer, who artfully brought the piece together.
- Designer Linda Wisner, who turned our words into exciting, easy-to-read pages.
- Artists Kate Pryka and Taylor Jean Engel, who made many concepts vividly visual.
- Image consultant Ethel Harms, who styled hair and makeup for our models.
- Copyeditor Ann Price Gosch, who fine-tuned the grammar and construction.
- McCall, Vogue, and Butterick pattern companies for sharing their beautiful fashion photography and fashion art to illustrate line, design, and color examples (for pattern information, see page 205).
- Students of Palmer/Pletsch sewing workshops, my image clients, those we met in a restaurant, members of a sewing guild, and friends or friends of friends who volunteered to be the "real people" examples for the book.
- Magnum Opus hair salon and Uptown EyeCare and Optical in Portland, Ore., for assistance with styling our models.

The information in these pages isn't new or revolutionary. It is time-tested and proven by artists and image consultants, many of whom have generously shared their knowledge through the years.

Looking Good ... Every Day is lovingly dedicated to my mother and to my "other mother" Edith, both of whom taught me to appreciate and value loveliness—external and internal—and to my daughters Mandi and Kate for continually pushing me to expand and freshen that appreciation.

For teaching tools when using the book as a text for image courses, contact the publisher.

Publisher's Cataloging-In-Publication Data
(Prepared by The Donohue Group, Inc.)

Nix-Rice, Nancy, author.
   Looking good ... every day : style solutions for real women / by Nancy Nix-Rice ; designed by Linda Wisner ; photography by Pati Palmer ; image consulting and styling by Ethel Harms ; illustration by Taylor Jean Engel and Kate Pryka ; editing by Pati Palmer ; copy editing by Ann Gosch.

   pages : illustrations ; cm

   "Palmer Pletsch publishing."
   Includes index.
   Issued also in various ebook formats.
   ISBN: 978-1-61847-040-9

   1. Women's clothing. 2. Fashion. 3. Color in clothing. 4. Beauty, Personal. I. Wisner, Linda, designer. II. Palmer, Pati, photographer, editor. III. Harms, Ethel, consultant. IV. Engel, Taylor Jean, illustrator. V. Pryka, Kate, illustrator. VI. Gosch, Ann, copy editor. VII. Title.

TT507 .N59 2014
646.34

NOTE: Whenever specific brands are mentioned, it is to save readers time by sharing products we have personally used and liked. Other items in the marketplace may be equally good.

print book ISBN: 978-1-61847-040-9
ebook ISBNs: PDF 978-1-61847-041-6; e-pub 978-1-61847-042-3; mobipocket 978-1-61847-043-0

Table of Contents

Foreword by Pati Palmer

Too many women start each day staring at a packed closet, moaning, "I have nothing to wear." Others spend the day worrying, "Does this make my rear end look fat?" or confessing sheepishy that they hate to shop.

Not surprising, considering the mountains of conflicting advice about dressing well—most of it from sources with their own agendas to promote:

♦ Retailers need to make sales, and it's easier to manage their inventory if women are convinced that certain items (like black dresses and white shirts) are "must-haves" for everyone.

♦ Magazines need to promote rapidly changing trends so that we need every issue to stay up to date.

♦ TV makeover shows need drama— can they make this week's candidate weep so we'll tune in for the next episode?

Looking Good ... Every Day has just one agenda: To provide real-life advice that regular women can apply regardless of their age, their dress size, their budget, or their personal style.

Clients and readers tell us that when they use these concepts they find that their wardrobes suddenly make sense. They shop more efficiently, buying better quality pieces without spending more. They coordinate countless outfits from a limited number of garments. They effortlessly walk out the door knowing they look good ... every day.

Of course, dressing well isn't one-size-fits-all. Each of us has a unique combination of characteristics, so your flattering choices won't be the same as your girlfriend's. But both of you can look and feel beautiful. The secret formula is "points of connection"—choosing style elements that echo the elements that already exist in YOU.

Along your personal style journey, be a skeptic. There is plenty of misinformation out there:

"They say…"
"Everybody should…"
"This season's Must-Haves are …"

Don't believe anything you hear about style— even this book—unless you can see the results with your own two eyes.

That's why *Looking Good ... Every Day* is packed with new photos and illustrations of style principles in action. Other images are drawn from our archives— because while specific styles come and go, design principles are timeless.

Culture and styles continually evolve. Today those timeless principles are viewed through the lens of more casual dress expectations, time-stressed lifestyles, and budget limitations. A creative young woman or her stylishly mature counterpart wants to adopt evolving trends, but only when those trends highlight the elements that are most beautiful about her own appearance.

Our original book, called simply *Looking Good,* published in 1996, became the textbook for training hundreds of new image consultants to help women look and feel beautiful. This new book reflects Nancy Nix-Rice's additional two decades of teaching image and ways to empower yourself to create that same transformation in your own closet.

Pati Palmer

Owner and CEO
Palmer/Pletsch Publishing

About the Author

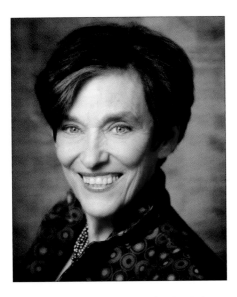

Nancy Nix-Rice is an image and wardrobe consultant, working with clients from homemakers and teachers to corporate executives and television personalities. Since 1989 she has transformed women's lives by transforming the contents of their closets. Nancy describes her private-client process as "a lot like that *What Not To Wear* show, but without the insults and power plays."

She also travels across the U.S. presenting workshops on appearance, and wardrobe for corporations, professional associations and women's conferences.

Over her 25-year career, Nancy has trained consultants for an international color and image company, served several terms as vice-president of the Association of Image Consultants International, edited AICI's member magazine *Image Update,* and garnered sales awards in a number of image-related companies including Beauty For All Seasons, Doncaster, Karla Jordan Jewelry, and CAbi clothing.

She was among the first to earn AICI's coveted "Certified Image Professional" certification. She also trained with the Professional Image Institute in Atlanta, and co-authored (with PII president Susan Bixler) *The New Professional Image—Business Casual to the Boardroom.*

Her earlier career—in the home sewing field—included managing and owning award-winning retail fabric stores, creating a top-ranked sewing school, managing the national consumer training programs for Baby Lock sewing machines, and appearing as sewing spokesperson on both QVC and the Home Shopping Network. She continues to write about sewing and wardrobe topics for *Sew News* and *Vogue Patterns* magazine, and to present educational programs for the American Sewing Guild and the Association of Sewing and Design Professionals.

Nancy is the mom of three adult children and five stepchildren. She and her husband, attorney Rob Litz, live in St. Louis and enjoy DIY home improvement projects and frequent travel.

Nancy is available for color and wardrobe consulting and presentations on style and wardrobe development. Complete contact information is listed on page 204.

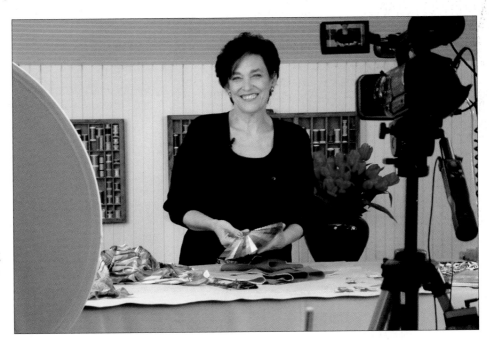

Nancy filming the Looking Good LIVE! *video.*

Why Bother Looking Good?

The Importance of Image

Our mothers—bless their hearts—love us for what we are on the inside. But the rest of the world assesses us based largely on appearance. We humans seem to have an inborn tendency to categorize others almost instantly, when appearance is the only input we have to consider.

Glance at the women below and notice the instantaneous assumptions you make about them.

♦ Which women look more confident?
♦ Which are more influential in the community?
♦ Which have more money? More education?
♦ Which have higher-level careers?
♦ Which travel to more exciting places?
♦ Which would turn heads?

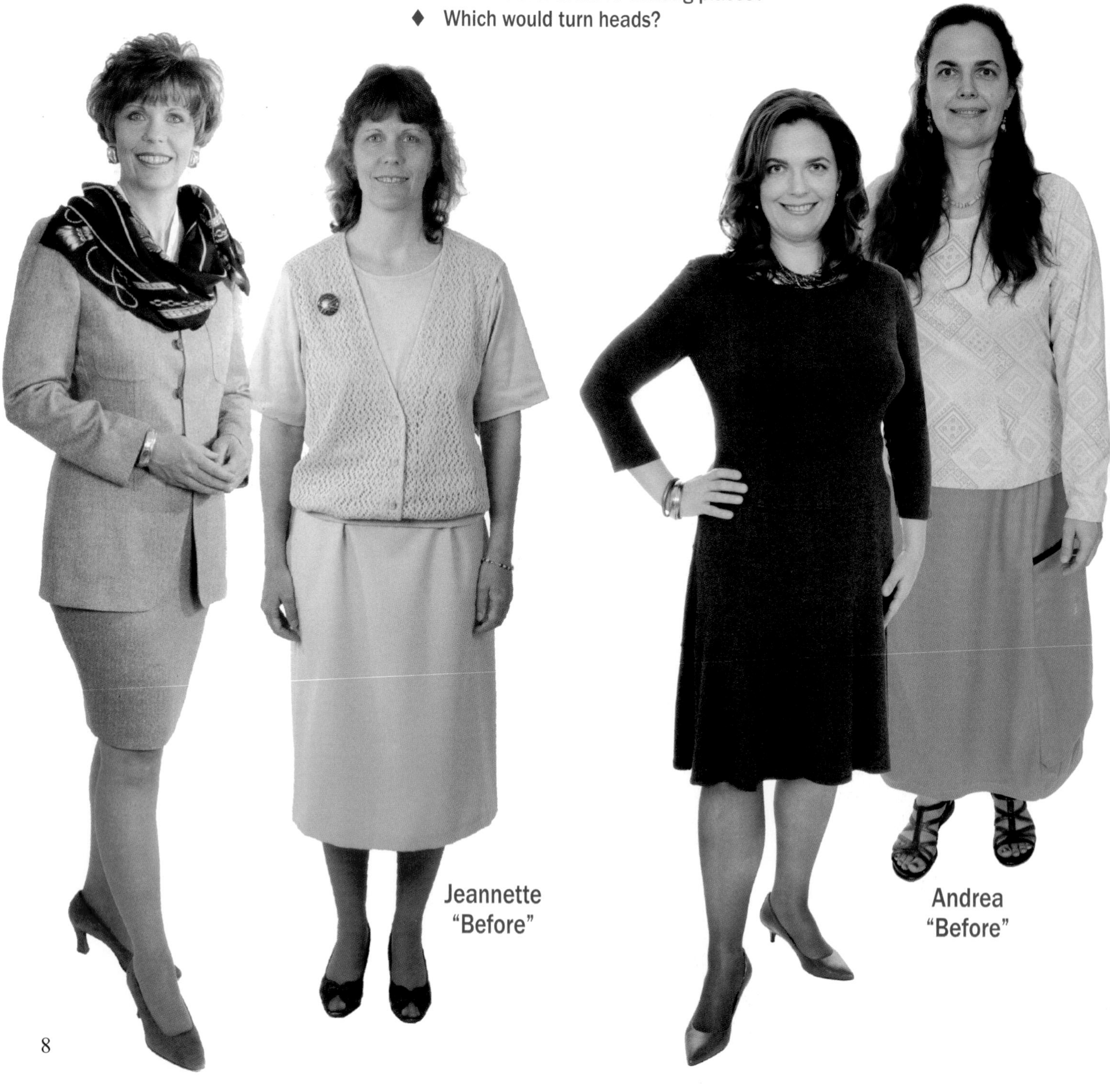

Jeannette
"Before"

Andrea
"Before"

Of course you're seeing before/after photos of three women. But differences in appearance cause most people to make vastly different assumptions about the "before" women and the "afters."

Even if you don't care one bit what other people think about you (really?), looking your best impacts your own confidence and self-concept.

The average American woman glimpses her own reflection 50 times each day. And each time, she instantly reacts with a mental "Ah, YES" or "Oh, NO!" What a confidence builder—or confidence destroyer—that can be.

So if appearances are that important, why don't we all look fabulous every day? We find that women have a pretty standard list of excuses:

♦ I'm too old…

♦ I'm too heavy…

♦ I'm too thin. (OK, we don't hear this one often)…

♦ I'm too short. Or too tall…

♦ I don't have time to shop…

♦ I don't have enough money…

♦ There is nothing in the stores for a person like me…

♦ I just don't know how to make flattering choices…

The only real reason is that last one—lack of know-how. When you apply the principles in this book you'll discover your own unique way of looking good ... every day, whatever your age, whatever your dress size, whatever your height, your schedule or your budget.

It isn't about the latest trend, the hot new designer, the pricey boutique or the outfit on the mannequin. It's all about discovering YOU and the styles that suit your visible characteristics and your inner essence.

As style icon Coco Chanel famously said, "Fashion is fleeting; style endures."

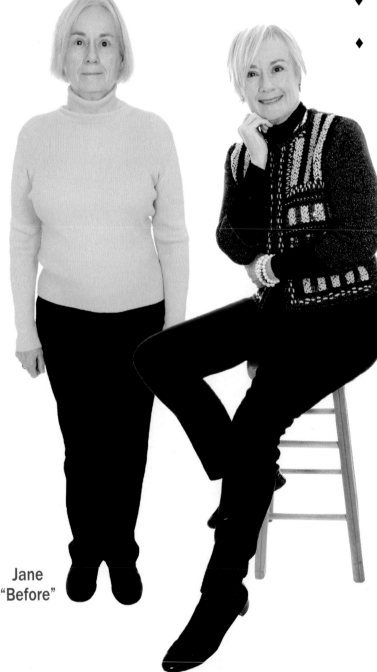

Jane
"Before"

Three Concepts

Before we launch into those timeless principles, there are three concepts you need to embrace:

1: You are beautiful.

Beautiful isn't one specific set of female characteristics, just as it isn't one specific flower or one specific sunset. There are infinite ways to be beautiful. The biggest wardrobe mistakes we see women make are attempts to hide what they consider flaws in their appearance. You may not love every characteristic that makes you YOU. But when you spotlight things you feel great about, everyone's attention will go to those, and your perceived challenges will fade into oblivion.

2: You are worth full price.

We females often seem programmed for bargain hunting. But a bunch of random items from the clearance rack usually add up to "nothing to wear." You're about to learn exactly what looks the very best on you. If you occasionally find one of those perfect items on sale—hooray! But the "perfect" part is much more important than the "on-sale" part. With the know-how you're about to gain, you can pay full price every time and still build a beautiful wardrobe on your current budget.

3: Focus on "points of connection."

The more characteristics that exist in common between YOU and the clothes and accessories you wear, the more lovely you will look. And as an added bonus, all those items will be connected with one another, taking the mystery out of mixing and matching. Look for colors, silhouettes, style details and accessories that repeat the elements of your own appearance and watch the magic happen.

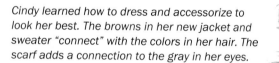

Cindy learned how to dress and accessorize to look her best. The browns in her new jacket and sweater "connect" with the colors in her hair. The scarf adds a connection to the gray in her eyes.

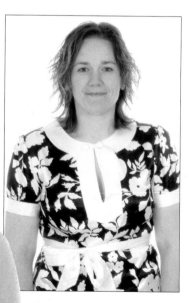

A blouse that doesn't harmonize with her coloring isn't a bargain at any price.

The Game Plan

The new *Looking Good...Every Day* is organized into three sections:

1. Chapters 1 through 8 train your eye to find points of connection between you and the clothes and accessories you choose.

2. Chapters 9 through 12 walk you through a step-by-step process of refining your wardrobe.

3. Chapters 13 through 19 bring you special reference information—makeup, fabric traits, clothing care, closet organization, custom sewing and alterations, travel tips and more.

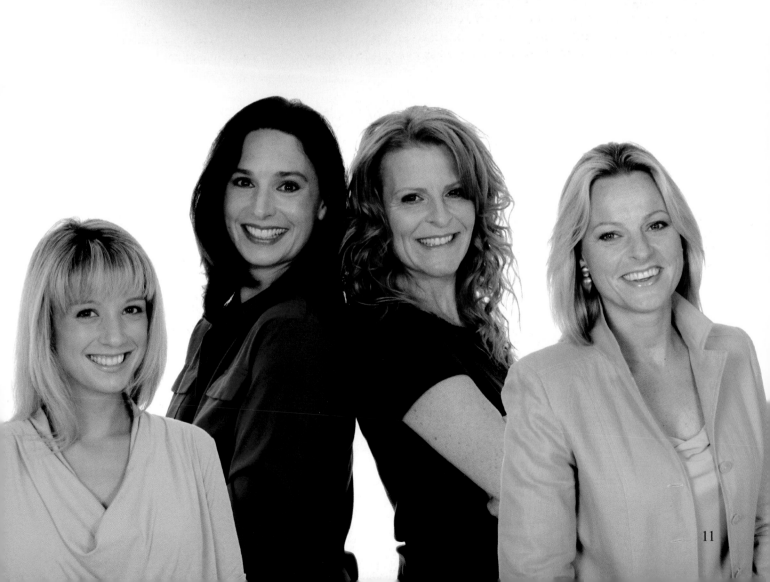

Chapter 1
Color Connections

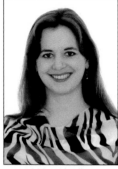
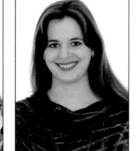
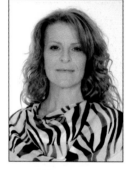
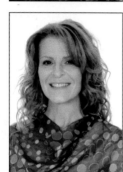
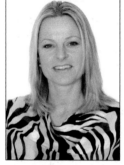
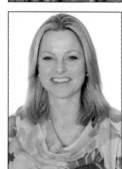
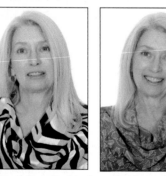

Fashion's favorite black-and-white color scheme is actually overpowering for most women. See how the focus moves from the stark, high-contrast print in the left-hand photos to the women's faces in the pictures on the right. Personalized color choices showcase their unique beauty...with or without makeup.

After decades of dressing women, we are convinced that the foundation for a flattering, versatile wardrobe is always the connection between the clothing and the client's personal color pattern.

In your best colors, you'll look beautiful, with glowing skin, rosy cheeks, sparkling eyes, and hair filled with highlights. But put on the opposite colors and immediately you'll look drained and tired, with blotchy skin, dull eyes and hair, even illusions of under-eye circles and double chins.

The great news is that this powerful appearance enhancer is absolutely FREE. It doesn't cost a penny more to buy that sweater in a color that makes you glow than to buy it in a color that makes you look like you died yesterday. And it doesn't take any longer to get dressed in the right colors than in wrong ones.

Some women are afraid that learning their best colors will be too limiting. But nearly every woman can wear nearly every color family. It's just a matter of determining the specific hue, value and intensity of blue or green or red that is most effective for her.

Knowing Your Best Colors Saves You Money

♦ The average American woman has at least $3,000 invested in her wardrobe. Just one or two outfits that hang unworn can be as costly as a color consultation.

♦ Defining your best colors eliminates impulse buying and makes you less likely to jump on a fad color that doesn't flatter you or go with anything in your closet. It helps you resist the "it was such a great markdown" method of color selection too.

♦ Consistently shopping with your best colors in mind creates a natural harmony within your wardrobe and leads to all sorts of happy accidents—wardrobe items that just seem to go together without conscious planning.

Points of Connection

So how do you know which colors are your personal best? You look for **"Points of Connection."**

Temperature Connection

The color wheel is a systematic representation of all the colors we see, organized according to the proportion of warm yellow pigment or cool blue pigment each color contains.

Just as colors can be classified as warm or cool based on the presence or absence of yellow pigment, humans can be described as warm or cool based on their unique body coloring.

The first step in pinpointing flattering colors is to echo the warmth or coolness of your personal coloring.

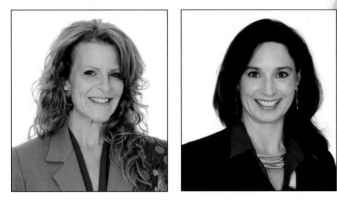

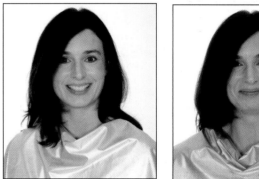

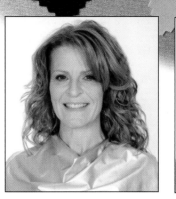

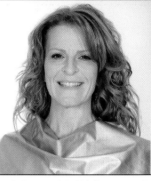

Your skin, hair and eyes will connect with colors that repeat your own temperature, causing a glowing appearance.

A Simple Test for Warm or Cool

On the most basic level, some women can determine their own temperature category—warm or cool—with this simple test. Hold sheets of gold and silver metallic paper or fabric alternately near your face. If the gold is obviously more harmonious, your undertones are WARM. If the silver is noticeably more flattering, your undertones are COOL.

The red-haired woman has WARM coloring that is enhanced by gold, and by golden-based colors. The dark-haired woman has COOL coloring that looks best with silver and with cooler, non-golden colors. (If you can't tell which is better on you, stay tuned. We'll explain why on page 17.)

Once you've determined your most enhancing metallic, you can hold that metal up next to a color you are considering for your wardrobe. If your metal looks good with the color, chances are the color has the right undertone for you.

There are more characteristics to consider, so this test doesn't pinpoint your very best colors. But it can steer you away from the range of colors that are drastically wrong for you.

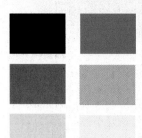

Value Connection

The next step in choosing optimal wardrobe colors is the element of value—how light (a tint) or how dark (a shade) the color is. Every color family exists in a range of values, arranged here from very dark to very light. You will look your best in colors whose value is close to the overall value of your personal color pattern.

Your personal value is determined by the combination of your skin, hair, and eyes. Blonde hair, porcelain skin, and pale blue eyes add up to a light/soft value. A woman of color, with rich brown skin, black hair, and brown eyes would be a dark/strong value. A high-contrast woman with pale to medium skin, dark eyes, and dark hair would also be classified as a dark/strong value.

Wearing colors that balance with your personal value pattern gives you a unified appearance from head to toe. (That allows you to look taller and trimmer in the bargain.) Wearing colors in a significantly mismatched value creates the effect that your head is somehow separate from the clothes and your body.

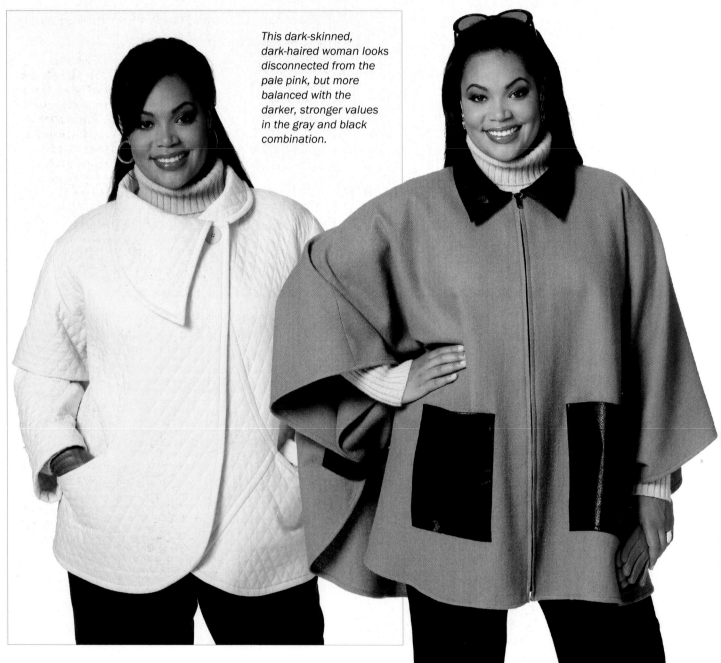

This dark-skinned, dark-haired woman looks disconnected from the pale pink, but more balanced with the darker, stronger values in the gray and black combination.

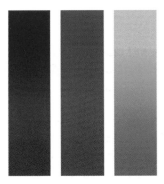

Three colors muted with their complement. (See page 19 for other examples of muting.)

Intensity Connection

Intensity refers to the clarity of a color—pure and saturated or more muted. A pure color becomes muted when it is blended with its complement (its color wheel opposite). It can also be muted by blending with brown or tan—a warm effect called toasting. Or it can be muted by blending with black or gray—a cool effect called silvering.

Characteristics like bright eyes or hair color, smooth skin and sleek hair texture can give a woman clearer, more intense coloring. Softer personal colors, more textural or multicolored hair, and eyes with varied highlights all contribute to a gentle, muted color pattern. The objective is to choose colors about as bright or as muted as your own color pattern.

Ironically, women with gentle, muted coloring often describe themselves as "drab" and try to brighten up their look by wearing overly bright colors. This approach actually makes their lovely, subtle coloring look dull by comparison. Surrounded by more muted wardrobe colors instead, their appearance takes on a natural glow.

Women with clear coloring, on the other hand, do look drab wearing muted colors; they need the connection of equally bright/clear clothing colors to showcase their beauty.

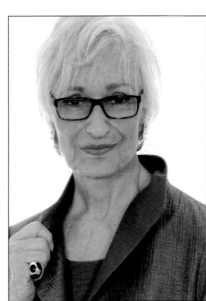

Ginni's clear coloring balances well with intense, saturated, clear colors like the royal blue on the left and looks dull with muted ones like the gray on the right.

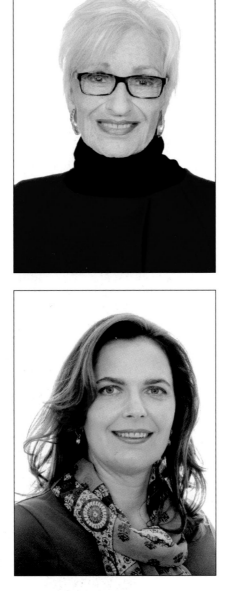

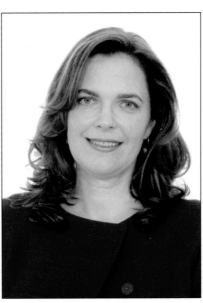

Andrea's muted coloring is showcased by muted fashion colors on the left, but overwhelmed by intense, clear ones like the blue jacket on the right. The grays in the printed scarf connect with the intensity of her gray eyes.

The "Four Seasons" of Color

The traditional "four seasons" approach considers temperature, value, and intensity as either/or concepts and combines them to create four categories. Winter and Spring, on the left, are bright. Summer and Fall, on the right, are more muted. The cooler women are at the top and warmer at the bottom.

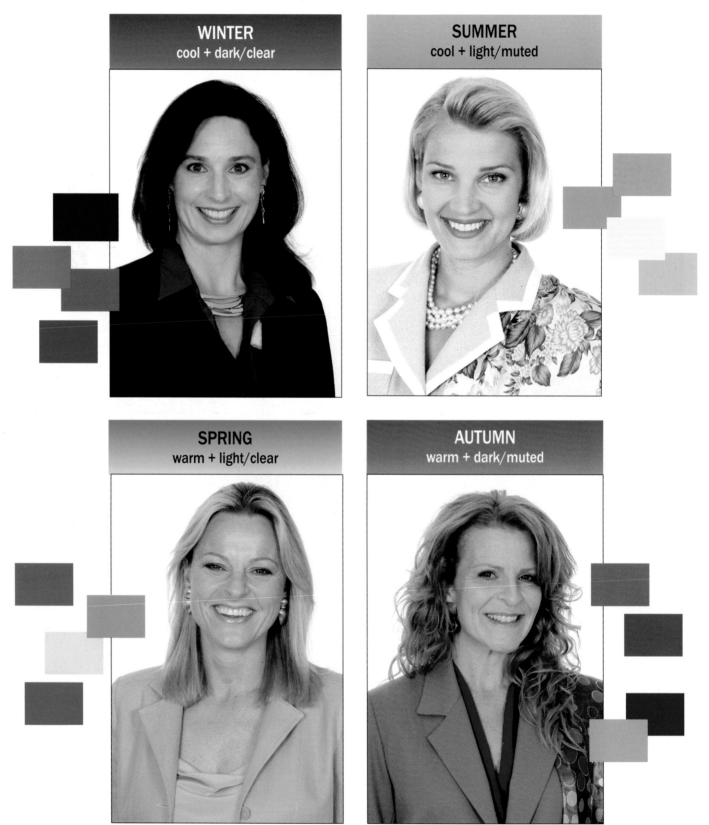

WINTER
cool + dark/clear

SUMMER
cool + light/muted

SPRING
warm + light/clear

AUTUMN
warm + dark/muted

Beyond Four Seasons

Some women fit into one of those seasonal stereotypes just beautifully. But many others do not. Why? Because color temperature, value, and intensity aren't really either/or concepts. Women can have color patterns along the entire continuum of each characteristic.

Variations of Warm and Cool

For example, the gold/silver test doesn't work for everyone because color temperature isn't an either/or trait. There are very warm women (the obviously gold gals), medium warms, barely warms, middle people, barely cools, medium cools and very cools (the decidedly silvers)—an infinite continuum of temperatures.

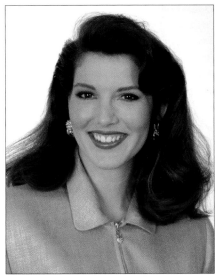

warmer

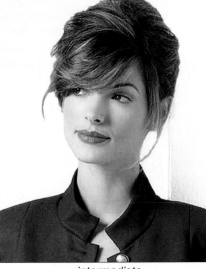

intermediate

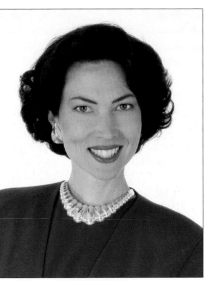

cooler

Similarly, nearly all fashion color families are also available in a continuum of temperatures. Left to right, these greens go from warm to cool.

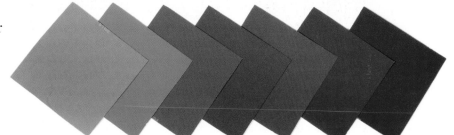

The mid-range colors below work with both gold and silver.

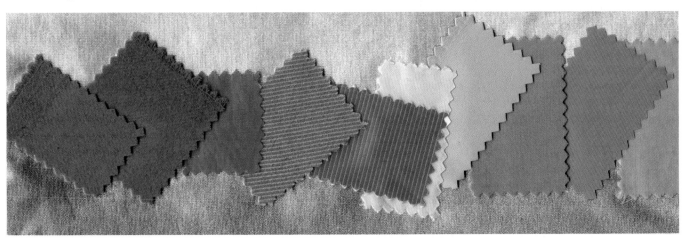

Variations in Value

The same concept applies to personal color value. Women can have very light coloring, medium light, mid-value, slightly dark and so on. Characteristics like stronger hair colors or darker eyes would influence your place along the continuum.

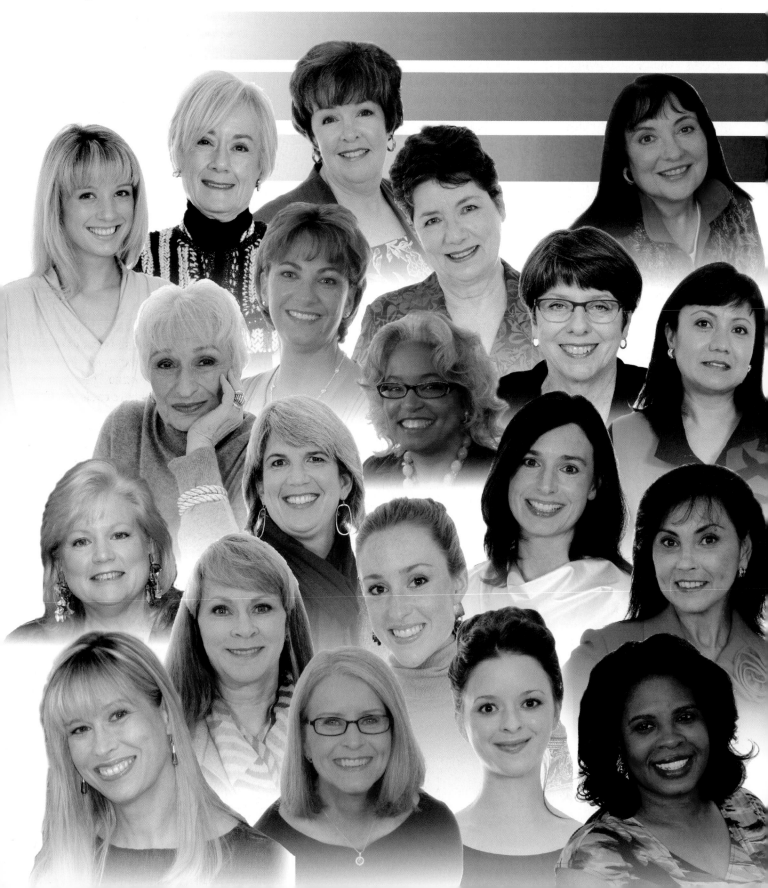

Variations in Intensity

The same kind of continuum exists for personal color intensity.

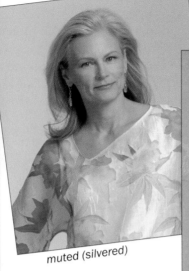

muted (silvered)

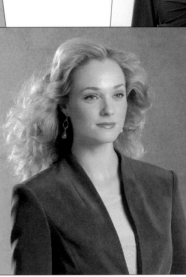

intermediate (toasted)

more clear

Summary

In a four seasons model, women with color characteristics that differ from the either/or extremes of warm/cool, light/dark or clear/muted were pushed to one side or the other of an artificial dividing line. That typically left them with seasonal color recommendations that weren't a great fit. Sometimes the same woman was placed in different categories by different consultants, depending on where each one drew that arbitrary line.

The most sophisticated approaches to color recognize an infinite number of personal color patterns. Highly trained consultants create recommendations that are uniquely personalized to each individual client's temperature, value, and intensity as well as the specific colors found in her skin, hair, and eyes.

For example, the women below might both be classified as Autumns in a seasonal system. But a customized analysis would distinguish subtle differences between their color patterns and create personalized color palettes for each of them.

complement   toasting   silvering

A pure color becomes muted when it is blended with its complement (its color wheel opposite). It can also be muted by blending with brown or tan—a warm effect called toasting. Or it can be muted by blending with black or gray—a cool effect called silvering. (The color squares below the strips show what was used to mute the blue.)

two very different "Autumns"

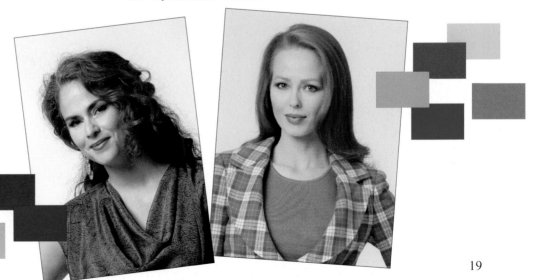

Coloring Changes With Age

As you mature, pigmentation diminishes and the colors of your skin, hair and eyes all soften. That reduces your color value and intensity. It can also make a warm woman appear more cool, since so much of her perceived warmth came from previously golden, red or auburn hair color.

Our graphic designer, Linda Wisner, has cool, soft, muted coloring. By age 45, she was wearing softer colors than she chose when her darker hair color gave her a stronger personal color pattern.

Linda today is even lighter in her hair color and, as a result, her palette has also changed a bit.

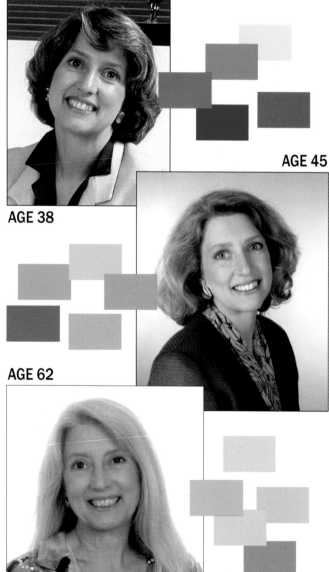

AGE 38

AGE 45

AGE 62

Do You Need a Professional Color Analysis?

Unless you happen to fit decisively into one of the four seasonal categories, a professional color analysis is one of the best investments you can make in your wardrobe. A trained professional can assess your coloring objectively, comparing you to a wide range of other women. She can give you pinpointed guidance on which colors to choose for your clothing and which ones to scrupulously avoid.

You'll especially want to consider a consultation if:

- ◆ You've never been analyzed before.
- ◆ Your previous four-season swatches don't seem to fit as well as they used to.
- ◆ Those old swatches are lying unused in a drawer; if they were serving you well you'd never shop without them.
- ◆ You were analyzed more than once, with different seasonal classifications.
- ◆ You have had a significant change in coloring (especially hair color) since your previous consultation.
- ◆ It's been more than 10 years since your previous analysis.

Choose your consultant carefully. Beyond the cost of the analysis itself, you'll spend countless dollars on clothing over the years, based on his or her recommendations. Here are some questions to ask before you schedule an appointment:

Q: What system do you use?

A top consultant uses a recognized system, not just her own personal opinions. She should be able to describe her philosophy and process in terms you understand.

Q: How were you trained?

Color analysis is NOT a read-the-book skill. Since it calls for making sophisticated visual comparisons, comprehensive hands-on training is essential.

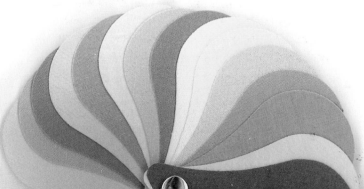

Q: Will we work in an individual session or a group?

A one-on-one consultation is obviously the most personalized and in-depth. However, a group of two or three participants can provide a good learning experience because you can see the color impact on another person much more objectively than on yourself. A large group—an adult education color class or a color "party"—doesn't allow personalized information for each participant. It can be a good introduction to color concepts and a chance to evaluate the ability of the instructor, should you decide to schedule a private session later.

Q: What lighting do you use?

Because light affects color to such a great degree, indirect natural daylight is the best choice. If your analysis will take place after dark, the artificial lighting should be carefully color-corrected to simulate daylight.

Q: Do I have to remove my makeup?

It is difficult to get an accurate analysis with your full makeup on because your current makeup may not be the best for your coloring. Even though it takes a little longer, removing it is an important step.

Q: What swatches will I receive?

You'll want fabric, printed, or painted swatches of the recommended colors to use as a permanent shopping reference. The number of swatches is important. Ten to 15 would be too limiting for most people; a hundred or more could be overwhelming. A range of 40-60 is about right for most people.

Q: What additional services are available?

Instruction in using your colors should be part of the basic consultation fee. Supporting print materials are a nice addition. Information about selecting compatible makeup colors is also important. (If the colors next to your face affect your appearance so dramatically, just imagine the impact of the colors ON your face.) Some color consultants carry their own line of cosmetics to help you make informed choices. Some consultants also offer closet audits, wardrobe planning, and personal shopping services to help you transition into your new color palette.

Q: How much will it cost?

As with most purchases, you get what you pay for. Expect to pay from $150 to $500 or more, depending on the area of the country. But you can save back the entire investment by avoiding just one or two costly shopping mistakes. A "free" color analysis at a home party or department store makeup counter can be a very costly mistake, since the consultant may be more thoroughly trained to sell you her products than to offer professional color advice.

Q: What if there is no color consultant in my area?

Some consultants offer color consultations via photographs for women who do not live near them. Verify the consultant's experience before you try this method, since it is more challenging than working face to face. The accuracy of the results depends entirely on the color accuracy of the photographs you provide. Take front and profile views in indirect natural light, then check carefully that the resulting prints match your true coloring. Don't try to save time by sending electronic files rather than hard-copy prints. The colors a consultant sees on her monitor may differ widely from the images you see on yours. However, technology keeps improving!

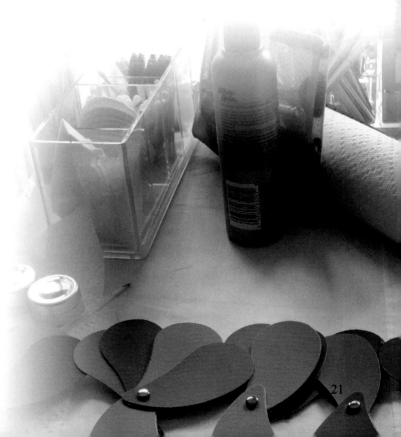

One Woman's Color Adventure

Cennetta, an expert seamstress and winner of the Palmer/Pletsch 2012 sewing contest, worked with color consultant Ethel Harms when she attended a Palmer/Pletsch workshop.

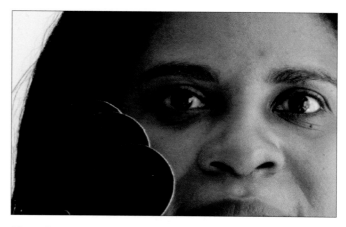

These browns match the colors in Cennetta's eyes.

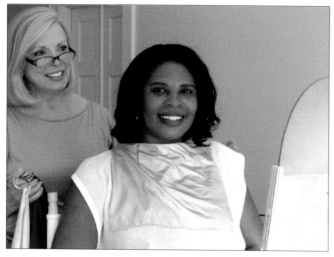

Ethel uses metallics to decide if Cennetta is warm or cool. Warm looks better.

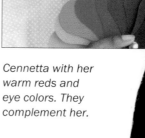

Cennetta with her warm reds and eye colors. They complement her.

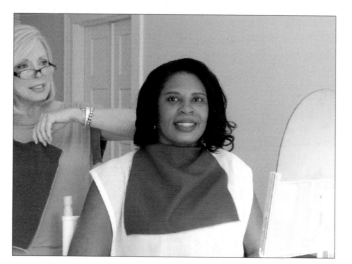

Warm red over blue red confirms it.

The complete color fan will include the most flattering choices from each color family.

22

Try Out Colors and Prints From Your Current Wardrobe

Of course your color analysis is only worth its cost if you USE it to develop a more flattering, versatile wardrobe. Few of us can afford to toss out our entire closet and start over from scratch. It can take a few seasons to develop a wardrobe totally keyed to your color fan, so be patient. Here's how to begin:

♦ Purge items that are polar-opposite wrong colors for you, especially if the items have other problems like poor fit or obvious wear and tear. You probably have at least twice as many clothes as you need anyway, so you'll do fine without those items.

♦ Resolve to make all new wardrobe purchases in your best colors.

♦ Items worn near your face matter most. If a suit is a less optimal color, try adding a blouse in your best shade. If a dress is the wrong color, wear a scarf or necklace in a flattering color. A touch of your hair color within the accessory adds to the flattery and visual connection.

♦ Don't overlook the option of dyeing an existing garment to a more flattering color for an instant update. See how-tos on page 191.

Try Out Colors and Prints Using Scarves

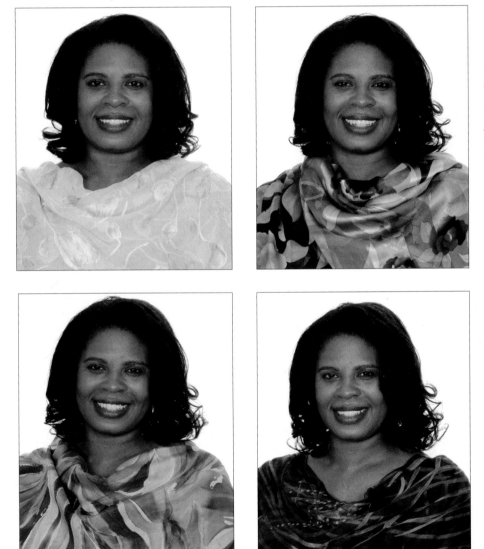

This pale print doesn't balance her strong coloring.

There is too much light gold in this print and some of the colors are too bright for her. Her golds are much richer like her personal coloring.

These clear colors are warm, but too light/bright/clear for her.

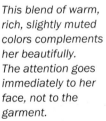

This blend of warm, rich, slightly muted colors complements her beautifully. The attention goes immediately to her face, not to the garment.

Shop With Your Colors

♦ Don't leave home without your colors—you never know when a shopping opportunity might develop.

♦ Compare garment colors to your swatches in daylight whenever possible, since some fluorescent lighting can distort colors.

♦ Understand that the colors you buy need to blend with your swatches, not necessarily match them exactly.

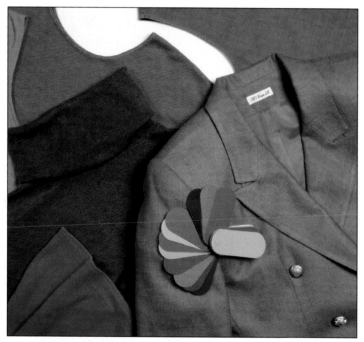

Up close, the tweed above has the same turquoise in it as the solid, but from a distance the two colors in the jacket visually blend, changing value to form a more muted blue that does not combine as well with the clear turquoise bottom.

♦ When considering a print or a pattern, look at the item from 8-10 feet away. The dominant colors—the ones you notice most from a distance—are the ones that need to match your swatches.

♦ Sometimes colors blend to form entirely new colors when viewed from a distance. Small prints, even in very bright colors, often look surprisingly muted from a few feet away. This is especially important when matching a print and a solid color you plan to wear together.

♦ When buying a recommended color you haven't worn before, consider trying it first in a smaller item like a scarf or T-shirt instead of a more expensive garment.

♦ Make sure you have your name and address on your color swatches; they can be expensive to replace.

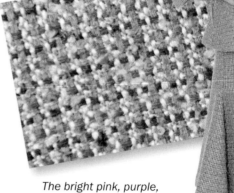

The bright pink, purple, and green in this tweed suit blend to appear almost neutral from a distance.

Color Your Cosmetics

Your color fan is a guide for choosing your most flattering makeup colors as well as wardrobe choices.

♦ Match foundation color to your natural skin tone.

♦ Choose lipstick, blush and nail colors in the various shades of red—pink, wine, peach, rust, coral, etc.—from your fan. Most women like to have a paler choice, a mid-tone, and a stronger option for lips and nails.

Since lip colors can look very different in the tube than they look on your face, test lipstick colors on your fingertips (the color of the skin is slightly darker there, much like the nude color of your lips), then compare the results to the red shades in your color fan.

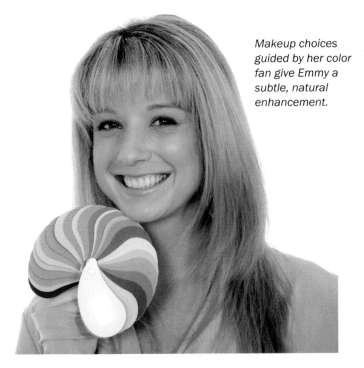

Makeup choices guided by her color fan give Emmy a subtle, natural enhancement.

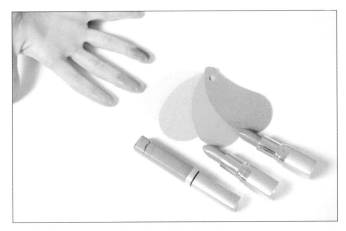

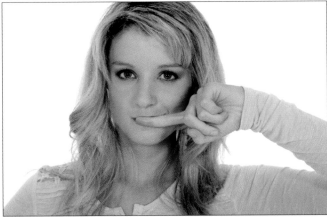

♦ Pick accent eye shadow colors that repeat your own eye color, or choose its complement (its color wheel opposite) instead. Emmy's gray eyes are emphasized by repeating subtle gray shades in her eye shadow.

♦ Use a dark version of your hair color for eyeliner and mascara. Brown mascara is far more natural looking than black on most blondes and redheads. It gives equal emphasis to the lashes without looking harsh and obviously artificial.

♦ Find complete makeup application how-tos on page 145.

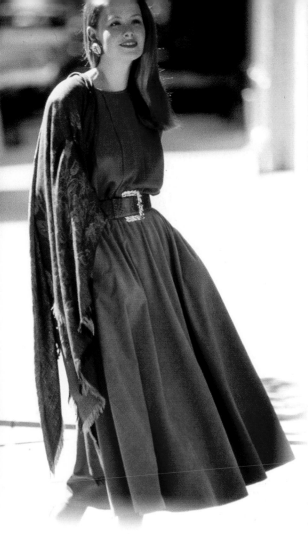

Neutrals – The Backbone of Your Wardrobe

These versatile colors will give you maximum fashion mileage because they can be worn over and over without being remembered.

Although retail and the fashion press work hard to sell us the myth that black is the universal neutral, it is actually flattering on only a small percentage of women. Variations in the brown family are more organic colors, much more likely to connect gracefully with organic human coloring.

Neutrals can be warm or cool; choose the ones that match your color temperature.

For a woman with lighter hair, the lowlight (darkest color strand) is her *Key Neutral*.

If there is no lowlight in your pale hair, go to a paint store and find a sample strip where the lightest color matches your hair. Then choose a color one or two shades darker on the same strip as a *Key Neutral*.

Navy can be an important neutral for almost any woman. Its cool versions range from dark and inky to softer and dustier. Its warmer versions lean slightly toward teal, much as the color of navy leather hints at the natural tan of the original hide.

COOL   WARM

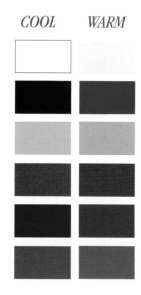

A **Key Neutral** for any woman is derived from her hair color.

For a dark-haired woman, her *Key Neutral* closely echoes her hair.

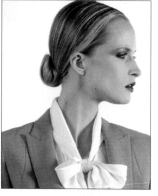

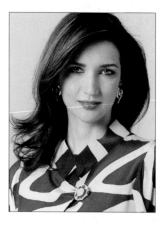

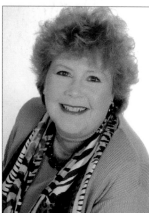

Select top-quality basic pieces like trousers, skirts, jackets and fine blouses or sweaters in your best neutrals. They will form the building blocks for a versatile wardrobe.

Combining Neutrals

An outfit in head-to-toe neutrals can be a sophisticated, elegant look if you avoid monotony by incorporating two of the following:

♦ Contrasts in light and dark values of the neutral.

♦ Interesting textures—tweed, mohair, brocade, lace.

♦ Interesting print or fabric surface.

♦ Unusual or dramatic garment design lines.

The Facts About Black

Understanding points of connection helps clarify why relatively few women really look their best in black. It just isn't part of most women's personal color schemes. The fashion and retail worlds have it as a universal "must have." Who knows why? But it certainly makes their business easier if all of us think we should be buying the very same thing.

Let's bust some black myths:

♦ **"Black makes you look thinner."** True, black is a receding—therefore minimizing—color. But no more so than other darks like chocolate brown, charcoal gray, and navy. And that whole advancing/receding concept is relative anyway. See page 34 for details.

♦ **"Black goes with everything."** Actually black goes with everything that goes with black— that is, mostly vibrant cool colors. Warmer, softer or silvered colors look harsh with black and more harmonious with warmer, softer or silvered neutrals.

Brick red, gold (warm), teal, and eggplant purple usually look better with brown.

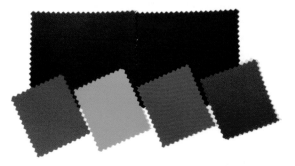

Cadet blue, mauve and lavender (cool) are more compatible with gray.

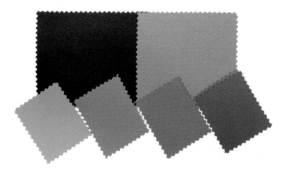

Soft, pale, warm colors are often better with camel shades.

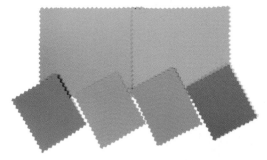

Soft, pale, cool colors are better with taupe shades or winter white.

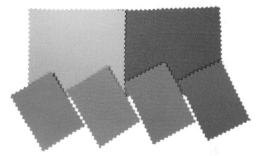

The most universal neutral is actually navy— picture it with all the colors above and see if you don't agree.

♦ **"All black clothes match."** Not so. You'll see blacks that are darker, others that are lighter, and others with a brownish or greenish tinge. Fiber content and surface texture also contribute to the variety of shades of black.

Because black is so prevalent in stores, most women have a closet full of black garments. See page 88 for ways to make them more flattering to your personal coloring.

The ecru shirt lets attention go to her face.

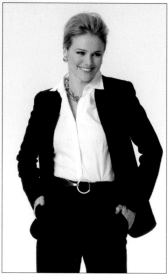

The bright white blouse draws attention to itself and away from the wearer.

The bright white in this print creates extreme contrast that dominates the entire look.

What About White?

The classic "must have" white shirt is another fashion myth, too bright to be flattering on all but a handful of women. Pearl, cream, whisper gray and barely blush are more flattering "whites" for most of us. Use them in the ways you formerly used bright white—blouses, shells, summer pants, bags and sandals for example.

Even these softened whites attract attention, so use them to spotlight an area you'd like people to notice. They can simultaneously distract the eye from another color or style element that's not so good for you.

Pay special attention to the shade of white in a print. Surrounded by other colors, even a soft white can easily appear brighter that it actually is, making the whole print too harsh and overpowering for a woman with warm or soft coloring.

The softer white in this floral doesn't overwhelm the wearer.

The many shades of "white."

Red

Everyone can wear some version of the red family, but it's not necessarily the fire-engine variety. If you have warm coloring, wear reds tinged with orange. Paler warm coloring? Try a softer orangey-red, toward peach. If you have cool coloring, wear blue-based cherry reds. Paler cool coloring is best in softer, dustier reds and pinks. And mid-temperature women glow in soft or vibrant shades of coral red.

The red family choices in your color palette are ideal guides for lipstick, blush and nail polish colors. You'll probably want to own three shades in those products to blend with your lightest, darkest and mid-value reds.

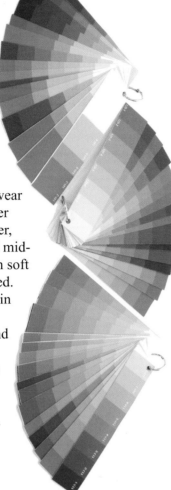

Palmer/Pletch sewing workshop attendee shopping for reds!

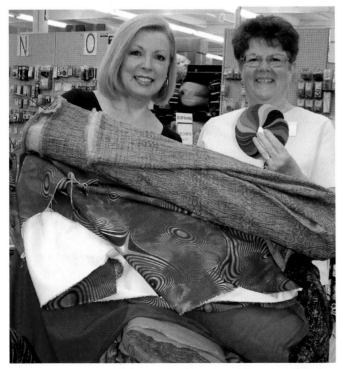

Your Body Essence Colors

Skin

The color of your skin is an effective, though nontraditional, pale neutral for shirts and sweaters, especially lovely in fabrics with subtle shine or surface texture. It can soften and feminize darker color schemes, making you seem more gentle and approachable. It's also the ideal choice for undergarments, eliminating any shadow-through by minimizing any color break between the garment and your actual skin.

Women of color can apply this principle using a paler version of their skin color—a soft camel or peachy-blush tone, for example.

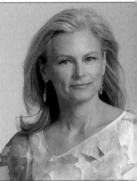

Hair

The colors in your hair work wonders to create visual unity between you and your clothing. Patterned clothes that include at least a bit of your hair color will create an unmistakable visual link to you. The effect is even stronger if the print motifs echo the shapes or texture of your hair.

Wearing earrings, a necklace, or scarf that includes this color is a great way to bridge between your face and a garment (even one in a less-connected color). Hair color is also a great choice for coats and for leather accessories —bags, belts and especially shoes. Since all your wardrobe color choices should look good with your hair color, it's just logical that hair-color accessories should look good with all those clothes.

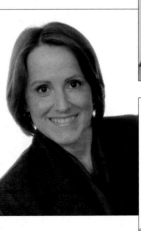

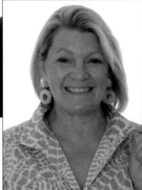

Eyes

The composite color of your eyes is an excellent choice to wear near your face. Use it for blouses and jackets, in earrings and necklaces, and as an eye shadow color. By repeating their color, you make your eyes a focal point in your overall appearance. This is a special benefit in one-on-one communications, where people will be compelled to make eye contact with you more readily and sustain eye contact longer.

Body Essence Intensifier Colors

Any color looks brighter and more intense when placed near its complement or color wheel opposite. You can use this technique to spotlight various elements of your personal color pattern.

Skin Intensifiers

Wearing the color wheel opposite of your skin color gives you a healthy glow. Since virtually all skin colors are variations of the warm red color family, intensifiers are typically shades of turquoise, aqua and teal. These colors can stand alone or add a spark of excitement to a neutral outfit. Wear them when you want to subtly stand out, not when you'd rather blend in.

Your specific intensifier is based on your exact color value and intensity, but it's hard for any shade from the turquoise/teal/aqua range to look bad on anyone. In fact, when you have to dress a group of people in matching garments, this color family is your safest choice. Consider it for bridesmaids' dresses, choir robes or other performance attire, and T-shirts for the family reunion.

Hair Intensifiers

When you wear the color wheel opposite of your hair color, your hair will take the spotlight, looking more lustrous and filled with highlights. Hair colors in the yellow range are intensified by purples. Reddish and auburn hair is intensified by rich greens and teal blues. Black or silver hair is called "achromatic" because it lacks color pigment. This ultra-cool hair is often intensified by bright royal or periwinkle blues.

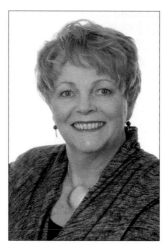

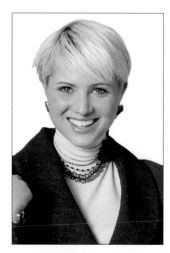

Eye Intensifiers

The color wheel opposite of your eye color provides an alternative way to spotlight your eyes. Wear it near your face in blouses, earrings, necklaces and scarves. Consider it in your makeup choices too—eye shadow colors or blushes and lip color. Blue-eyed

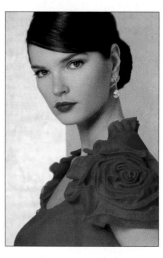

women often avoid stronger lip colors because they want their eyes to be a focal point, but actually the contrast of lipstick from your personal version of the red family makes blue eyes pop. Green eyes can be intensified by reds as well, or by plum clothing and eye shadow colors that emphasize their golden accents in the eyes. Brown eyes also look more golden when accented with plum shades.

Combining Colors

Nearly any two colors in your palette can be used together in a great outfit. If the mix is unexpected, so much the better. People will be dazzled by your creativity, as long as you include a link in the ensemble. A link is a multicolored accessory—a scarf or necklace is an obvious option—that incorporates both garment colors into one item. (See page 118.) It clearly tells the viewer that this is a planned outfit—not just the only pieces you had clean today.

Guidelines for Color Mixing

♦ **In a multiple color ensemble, choose a major amount of one color** (the suit, for example) and a secondary amount of another color (blouse). Introduce a third color, if you want, in a minor amount (shoes and belt perhaps). Equal amounts of two colors usually create an awkward balance.

♦ **The easiest color schemes are:**
- Neutrals head to toe.
- Neutral with a single color accent (blouse or accessories perhaps).
- Monochromatic—lighter and darker versions of the same color.
- Multicolor print or pattern worn with one of its component colors.

neutral head to toe   neutrals with a single color accent   monochromatic   multicolor print with component color

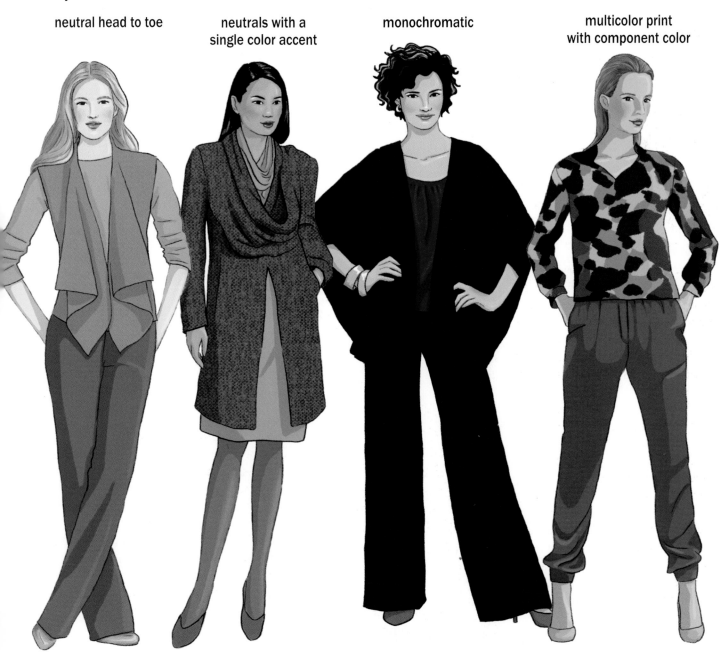

More Combinations

The color wheel can suggest more interesting color combinations for creative wardrobes. Some of these color schemes work best with palettes that are somewhat muted. Bright blue and orange suggest a high school marching band, while a rich navy accented with coppery rust exudes a cozy sophistication.

Primary colors—red, yellow, blue—are used to make all the other colors on the color wheel.

Secondary colors—orange, green, violet—are mixtures of two primary colors.

Tertiary colors—red-orange, yellow-orange, yellow-green, blue-green, blue-violet, red-violet—are mixtures of one primary and one secondary color.

Complementary color schemes combine colors that are color wheel opposites. Red/green, yellow/purple, blue/orange are examples. Use the two colors in deep or muted tones and unequal amounts.

Split-complementary scheme takes the colors on either side of the original color's complement. For example, start with the blue/orange scheme described above, then substitute red-orange and yellow-orange as the split-complements.

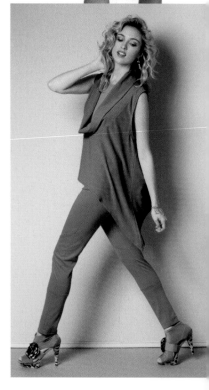

Analogous color schemes use three colors adjacent on the color wheel. Starting with the yellow-green from this print skirt, its analogous colors are yellow on one side and green on the other. A green suit with a yellow blouse and yellow-green accessories is an analogous color scheme.

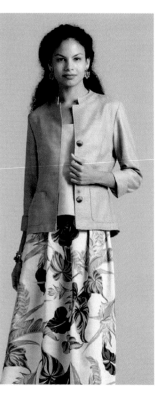

Triadic colors are linked by an equal triangle on the color wheel. They are the most challenging to combine, but can be striking when done well. Let one color dominate, and use the others as smaller accent areas.

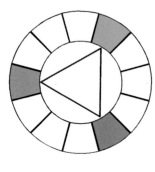

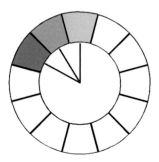

Color Contrast

Be cautious about mixing colors—even two choices from your color fan—that create a level of color contrast greater than the light/dark contrast in your personal color pattern.

Light/dark or bright/dark contrast is a magnet for attention. When the outfit is more contrasting than you are, all the attention goes to the clothes rather than to you. That's why black/white garments are so visually commanding in the retail environment—and why they are flattering to such a tiny percentage of women.

It is almost never effective to wear a contrast level greater than your own. Most women look their very best in a contrast level that approximates the personal contrast they see in the mirror.

Evaluate contrast by trying on the outfit, standing 5-10 feet from a mirror and squinting at the image. If the clothes pull attention away from your face, the contrast level is too extreme.

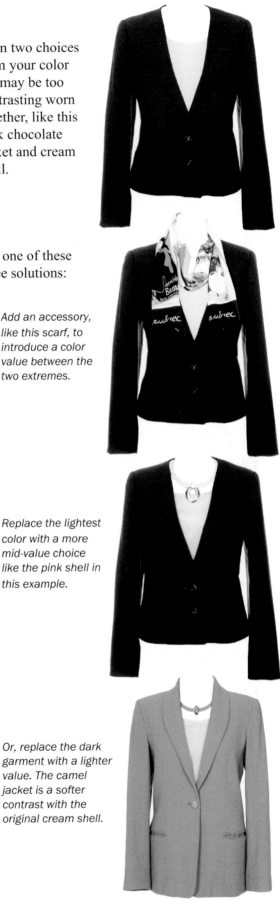

Even two choices from your color fan may be too contrasting worn together, like this dark chocolate jacket and cream shell.

Try one of these three solutions:

♦ *Add an accessory, like this scarf, to introduce a color value between the two extremes.*

♦ *Replace the lightest color with a more mid-value choice like the pink shell in this example.*

♦ *Or, replace the dark garment with a lighter value. The camel jacket is a softer contrast with the original cream shell.*

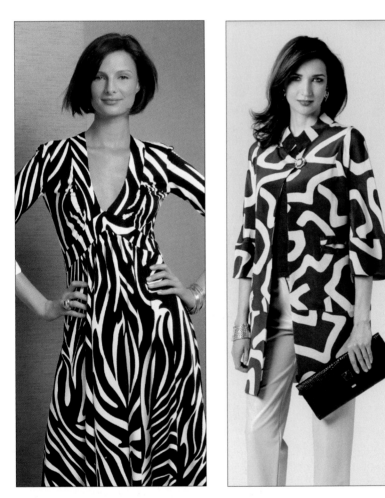

The dress on the left is too high-contrast and draws the eye away from the woman's face. The jacket on the right features a contrast level balanced to the coloring of the woman wearing it.

Advancing/Receding Colors

Color placement can dramatically affect visual body proportions. See how the yellow circle looks larger than the purple one in the diagram below.

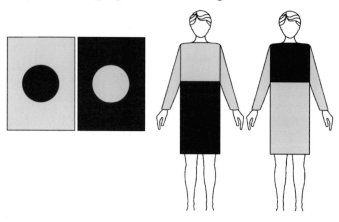

You can use color placement to give the illusion of a more balanced figure. Areas of lighter color enlarge and draw attention; areas of darker color minimize.

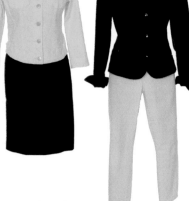

♦ Lighter, brighter, warmer colors and shiny surface textures all seem to move toward the viewer's eye, making the body areas they cover appear larger. Use them to emphasize areas you want to spotlight or to proportionally increase smaller body areas.

♦ Darker, cooler and more muted colors and matte surface textures all recede, making areas they cover seem smaller. Use them to let attention flow away from body areas you'd prefer to minimize.

Also notice how your attention goes to the places in the diagrams and photos where the color changes from light to dark. A "color break" is an attention magnet, so be sure to position one only at body points you want to emphasize.

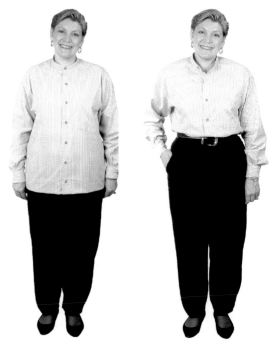

Pati was amazed that she looked slimmer with the top tucked in!

It's important to understand that advancing/receding color is a relative concept. You can't wear head-to-toe black and automatically look like a size 2. But within any fashion color scheme, you can position the more receding color to make the area it covers appear relatively smaller. In fact the very same color can either advance or recede, depending on the color it's combined with.

The same rust color advances when combined with dark brown, but recedes when combined with bright gold.

The Emotional Impact of Color

Although individuals may react differently to colors based on personal preferences and unique life experiences, numerous studies confirm that the majority of people often make certain color associations, such as:

- Black – powerful, strong, commanding
- Gray – conventional, elegant
- White – pure, precise
- Red – aggressive, dominant, dynamic, passionate
- Orange – distressing, stimulating, exciting
- Yellow – cheerful, stimulating
- Green – refreshing, natural, calming
- Blue – calming, comforting, soothing

Because color symbolism is often very culture-specific, these attributes can vary in different areas of the world. But psychological messages of color can be an important consideration, especially in business settings.

...tography compliments of the McCall Pattern Company. For a complete pattern listing, see page 204.

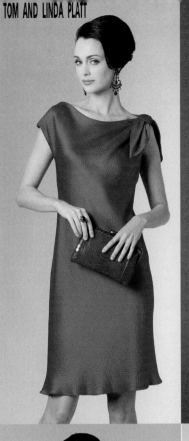

TOM AND LINDA PLATT

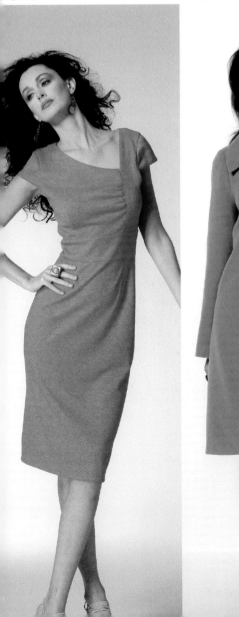

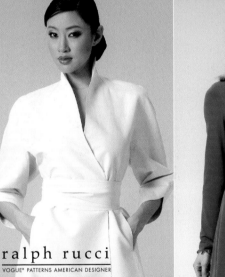

ralph rucci
VOGUE® PATTERNS AMERICAN DESIGNER

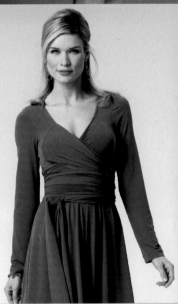

ANNE KLEIN

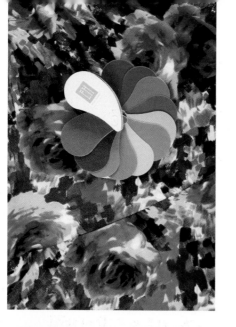

Here are three prints that work well for Marta.

Nearly a dozen blues and greens from Marta's color fan appear in this watercolor floral.

This batik echoes her rich, cool hair and eye colors.

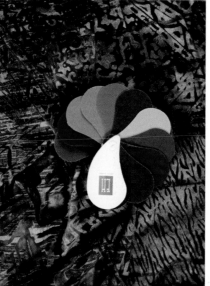

The prevalence of her best reds in this butterfly print outweighs the small amount of warmer peach and orange.

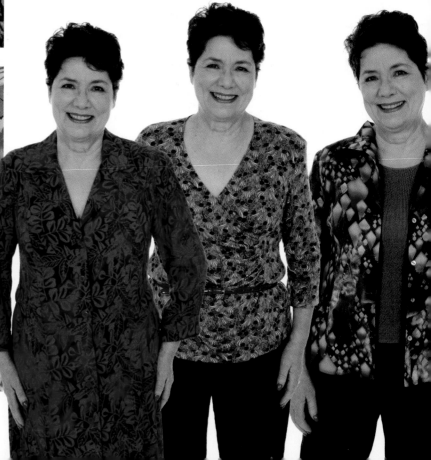

Choosing Print Colors

Because prints and other patterned fabrics (plaids, brocades) are so eye-catching, it is particularly important that they work well with your personal color pattern. Prints typically function much like an advancing color within an outfit, so use them most often on body areas you'd like people to notice, not ones you'd rather minimize.

Evaluate the color mix of a print by checking for these factors:

♦ **Individual colors that are in your color fan.**
Evaluate this from a distance, because the eye blends small areas of color, just like mixing paint pigments to form new shades.

♦ **Overall color *temperature* that matches yours.**
Checking the print with your best metallic is one good way to verify this. If you have cool coloring, watch out for even a small amount of colors like yellow, gold, orange or camel in a print. It takes only a small amount of warm color to raise the temperature of an otherwise cool color combination. Oddly, this principle almost never works in reverse. Adding a cool color to an overall warm mix doesn't do much to cool the overall look.

Marta's best makeup shades blend easily with the cool reds in the two prints below...

...but clash with the warmer orangey reds in this one.

36

◆ **Overall color *value* that matches yours.** Compare it to your entire color fan, or hold it up against your body and check in the mirror that it makes a unified visual picture with your face and hair.

◆ **Overall intensity that matches yours.** Soft colors and blurred motifs work with muted personal coloring. Bolder colors and distinct, outlined motifs work with bright personal coloring. Check in the mirror and ask yourself if you are wearing the print, or if it is wearing you.

◆ **No pale neutrals brighter than your best "white."** Even your best softened white can look too bright when it is surrounded by other colors in a print, so check this factor with extra care.

◆ **Reds, if any, that match those in your color fan.** Other reds in the print will make it challenging to select makeup. Do you choose lip and cheek colors that flatter your face but clash with the print, or ones that match the print but don't flatter your facial coloring?

◆ **Includes a touch of your hair color.** Although not an absolute requirement, the presence of your hair color makes an instant, and almost always flattering, connection between the print and you. That link is even stronger if the shapes in the print echo the textural aspect of your hair.

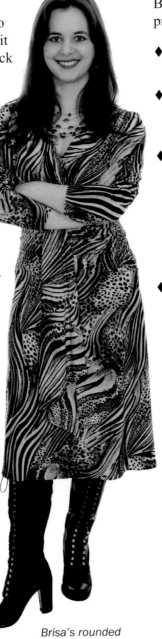

Brisa's rounded swirly print mimics the roundness of her features.

Beyond color considerations, your most flattering prints will have:

◆ **Shapes that echo the curve/angularity of your facial features** (see page 76).

◆ **Motifs in a scale that harmonizes with your body.** (See page 46). Some women use the size of their palm to define the largest motif they wear.

◆ **Print scale isn't just the size of the repeat,** however. Motifs appear larger when they are spaced apart on a solid background, and seem smaller when they are placed closer together. Motifs also look smaller when the larger design is made up of smaller components or when the colors are variegated rather than solid.

◆ **Motifs also seem smaller when they are sewn into draped styles** because the folds of fabric obscure the edges of the print shapes. The same print that might seem too big for you in a sheath dress could work fine in a softly gathered skirt.

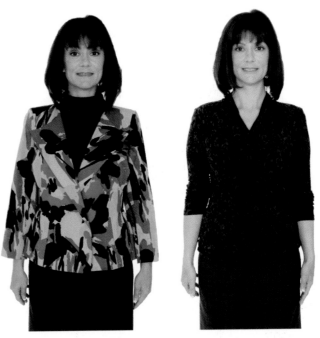

Tara is petite and is better in the smaller brown print than in the large multicolor print.

A flattering print can be a great starting point for a wardrobe grouping. If you like the colors together in the print, you'll almost certainly like those same colors in solid garments to mix and match. And the print piece can act as a link, unifying those additional solid pieces into understandable outfits. Read more about links on page 31 and 118.

CHAPTER 2
Silhouette Connections

A *Glamour* magazine survey confirms what we've long suspected: Over 95% of American women are dissatisfied with some element of their body proportions. That often-unjustified dissatisfaction makes it hard for women to objectively evaluate their body type and choose garments that will flatter them. In fact, the biggest style mistakes we see are usually the results of women trying to hide some imagined figure flaws.

Make a Body Graph

A "body graph" is a quick, fun and simple way to identify your shape and proportions regardless of your height. Palmer/Pletsch has tested and fine-tuned the steps of making a body graph with students in their workshops.

Though two people can make a body graph, as shown by Emmy and Lauren on the next pages, it is easiest to do in groups of four—one being graphed, one holding a ruler, and one marking while another stands back to make sure the pencil is perpendicular to the wall. Make it a party (or, if you are a teacher, a class you could teach).

Preparation

1. Cut newsprint or butcher paper* wider and taller than you are. (Tape two widths together if the paper is too narrow.) Fold it in half lengthwise and crease. Mark the foldline using a pen and yardstick.

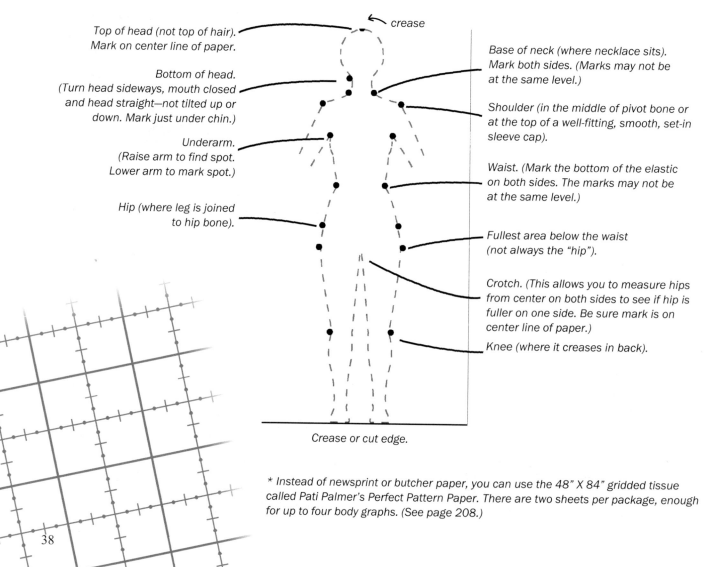

← crease

Top of head (not top of hair). Mark on center line of paper.

Bottom of head. (Turn head sideways, mouth closed and head straight—not tilted up or down. Mark just under chin.)

Underarm. (Raise arm to find spot. Lower arm to mark spot.)

Hip (where leg is joined to hip bone).

Base of neck (where necklace sits). Mark both sides. (Marks may not be at the same level.)

Shoulder (in the middle of pivot bone or at the top of a well-fitting, smooth, set-in sleeve cap).

Waist. (Mark the bottom of the elastic on both sides. The marks may not be at the same level.)

Fullest area below the waist (not always the "hip").

Crotch. (This allows you to measure hips from center on both sides to see if hip is fuller on one side. Be sure mark is on center line of paper.)

Knee (where it creases in back).

Crease or cut edge.

* *Instead of newsprint or butcher paper, you can use the 48" X 84" gridded tissue called Pati Palmer's Perfect Pattern Paper. There are two sheets per package, enough for up to four body graphs. (See page 208.)*

2. Tape the paper to a wall. Cut or crease the paper even with an uncarpeted floor.

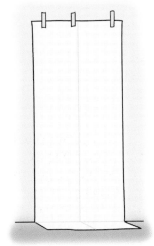

3. Wear nonbinding underwear or leotard and no shoes. Pin elastic around your waist—the bottom of the elastic is at your waist. Wear a chain necklace to mark the base of your neck.

4. Stand with your back against the paper in normal posture, centering your body along the vertical crease. Mark the top of head and crotch first to make sure you are centered on the fold. Look straight ahead. DO NOT LOOK UP OR DOWN!

5. Have a friend plot the points shown in the illustration on the previous page, using a new, long pencil and a nonflexing yardstick. Have her keep the yardstick close to your body, holding the opposite end so the entire yardstick is perpendicular to the wall. Then have her mark the paper at the edge of the yardstick that is next to your body.

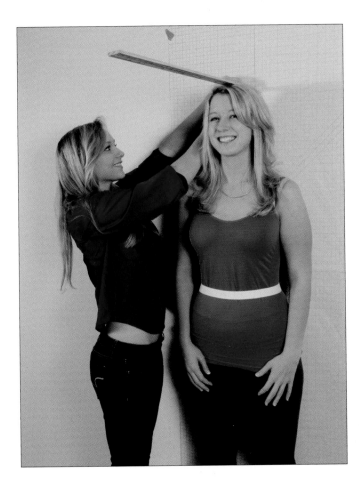

Step 1: Top of Head

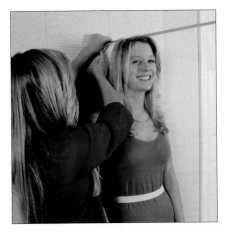

Make sure your head is centered on the fold and the ruler is perpendicular to the wall, firmly on top of your head, not hair. Mark the top of the head.

TIP: From the side view you can easily see if the ruler is perpendicular to the wall and parallel to the floor.

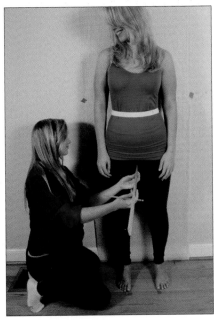

Step 2: Crotch

Mark the crotch to make sure your entire body is centered on the foldline. Put the ruler up close to body.

Step away and mark. Not only does this marking ensure you are centered on the foldline, it also allows you to measure each half of your body to see if your hip is fuller on one side than on the other.

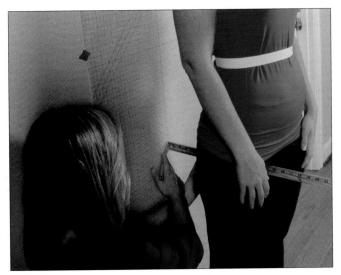

Step 3: Bottom of Head

Turn head sideways, mouth closed and head straight—not up or down. Mark just under chin. This determines head size in proportion to the rest of your body.

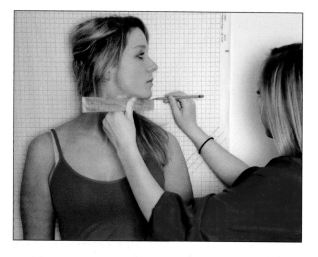

Step 4: Base of Neck

Mark base of neck on both sides where necklace sits. Marks may not be at the same level, depending on the curvature of your neck and slope of each shoulder.

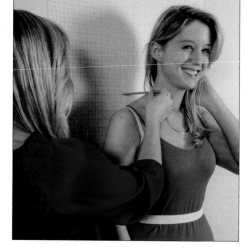

Step 5: Shoulders

Mark the point on the top of the shoulder where the arm pivots (the top of a fitted, set-in sleeve cap).

pivot point

Lower edge of set-in sleeve follows the "crease."

Step 6: Underarm

Raise arm to find the spot. Lower arm to mark the spot using a ruler and pencil, or pencil alone if you can keep the pencil perpendicular to the wall under your arm.

Remember to mark both sides.

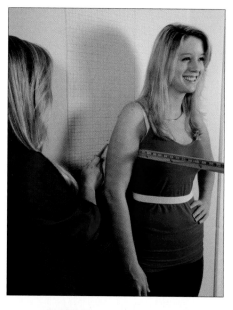

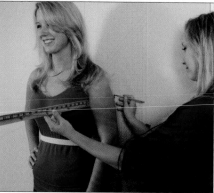

Step 7: Waist

Mark the *bottom* of the elastic on both sides.

HINT: The waist is generally at the top of the hip bone where you bend when you lean to the side.

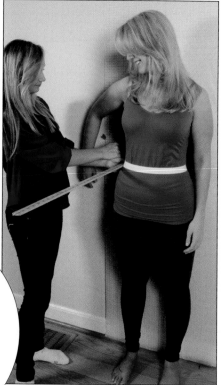

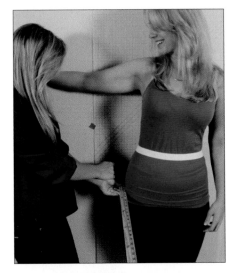

Step 8: Hip

Mark where leg is joined to hip bone—where you crease when you raise your leg to the side. The hip is not necessarily the fullest part below your waist.

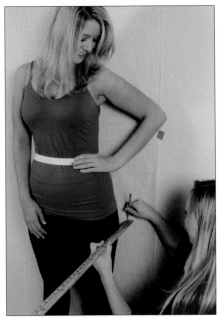

Step 9: Fullest Hip

This could be *any* area below your waist such as your high hip, hip, or thigh.

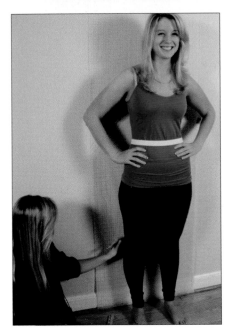

Step 10: Knee

Mark where knee creases in the back when you bend it.

Step 11: Trace Silhouette

Have a friend trace around your silhouette, connecting the dots to create your shape. Start at the neck. For accuracy the pencil must be perpendicular to the wall. Hold it with two hands. This helps you double-check the accuracy of your dots. If any marks appear to be off, check and remark if necessary.

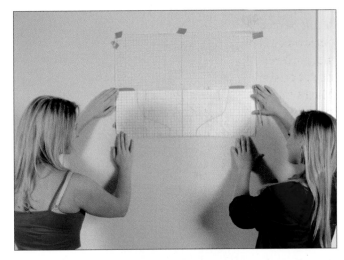

wall

Hold the pencil perpendicular to the wall.

Step 12: Step Away

Step away. With paper still taped to wall, fold it in half, matching the bottom of your feet with the top of your head. Fold it in half again and then again, creasing it into eight equal sections.

Unfold the paper and mark the fold lines with a permanent marker. (NOTE: We put poster board under the tissue so we wouldn't mark the wall.)

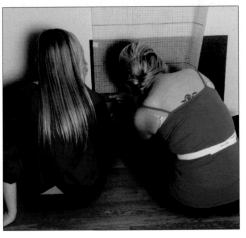

You can also use the marker to go over the pencil lines outlining your body to make your body graph show up better.

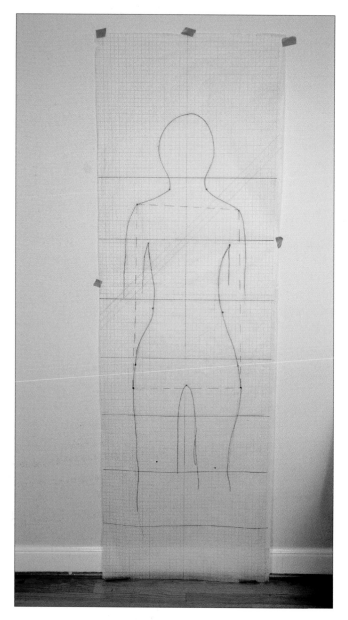

Step 13: Draw Line from the Neck Out

Draw a straight line from the base of the neck in both directions to above the shoulder dots, parallel to the nearest foldline. If dots are uneven, use the highest dot.

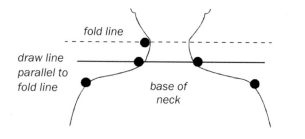

Step 14: Connect Shoulder to Hip

Draw a dotted line box that connects your shoulder dots to the fullest hip area dots.

Fullest hip area may be low in thigh area

...or it may be just below the waist.

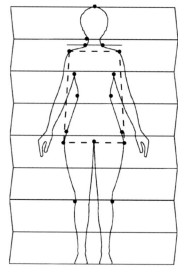
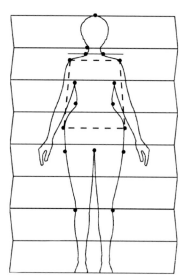

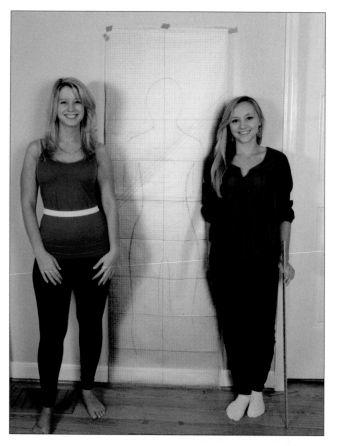

Note: The average figure is eight heads tall. The "ideally" proportioned body is divided as shown in the illustration on page 44.

Step 15: Identify Your Predominant Silhouette

Now examine the box around your torso. You will see not only your proportions, but the essence of your shape. Once your "outside line" is determined, the clothing that will fit you best will have similar outside lines.

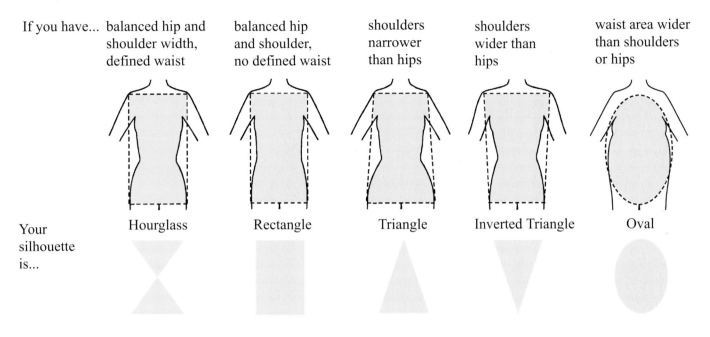

If you have...	balanced hip and shoulder width, defined waist	balanced hip and shoulder, no defined waist	shoulders narrower than hips	shoulders wider than hips	waist area wider than shoulders or hips
Your silhouette is...	Hourglass	Rectangle	Triangle	Inverted Triangle	Oval

Note that all but the Oval can be a little hourglass in their shape. For example, we might say you are a triangle with a hint of hourglass.

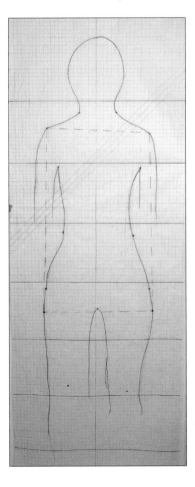

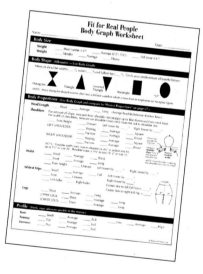

Step 16: Analyze Your Body

Now analyze your body, comparing your shape to the "ideal" proportions on the next page. Then fill out the Body Graph Worksheet on page 45. (If you prefer, make a photocopy of the page.) The box around Emmy's torso is a rectangle because her hip and shoulders are the same width. Her torso is a very, very slight triangle because her hip is wider than her shoulders.

Because the total difference is only 1", we will dub her as an hourglass. She is a little long-waisted and the hip line that can divide the body in half is below the middle line, so her upper half is a little longer than the lower half.

Compare Yourself to "Ideal" Proportions

Although no one is perfect, you have to start somewhere to have a point of comparison.

"Ideal" Proportions

Width from neck base dot out to shoulder dot is 4¾" for a pattern size* 10, up to 5¼" for size 20.

Shoulders slope 1 5/8" from neck base if you are a pattern size* 10, up to 2" for a size 20.

Underarm is halfway between top of head and hip.

Waist is halfway between underarm and hip.

Hip where leg is joined divides body in half.

Hips are 1" narrower than shoulders for garments to fall freely over hips.

Knee is halfway between hip and feet.

Soles of feet.

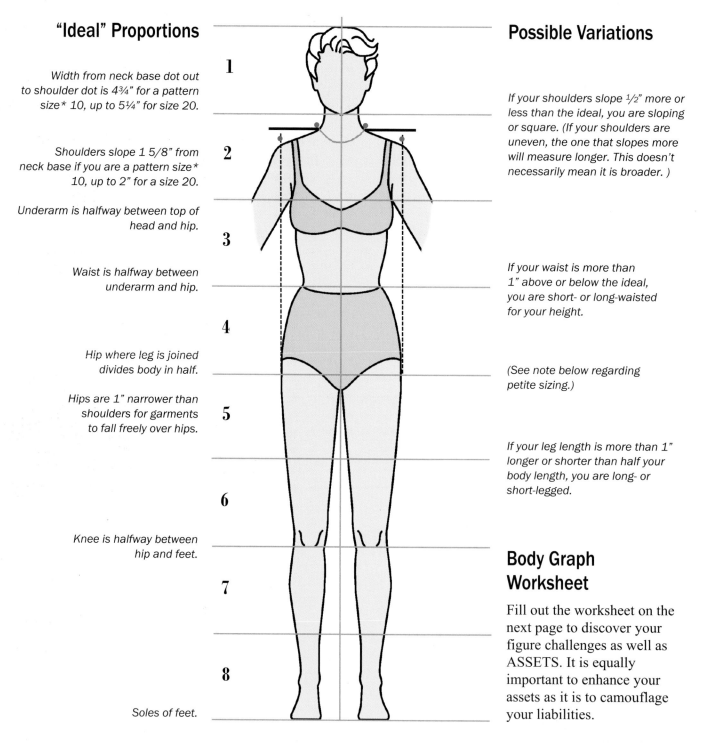

Possible Variations

If your shoulders slope ½" more or less than the ideal, you are sloping or square. (If your shoulders are uneven, the one that slopes more will measure longer. This doesn't necessarily mean it is broader.)

If your waist is more than 1" above or below the ideal, you are short- or long-waisted for your height.

(See note below regarding petite sizing.)

If your leg length is more than 1" longer or shorter than half your body length, you are long- or short-legged.

Body Graph Worksheet

Fill out the worksheet on the next page to discover your figure challenges as well as ASSETS. It is equally important to enhance your assets as it is to camouflage your liabilities.

*For more about proportions and using them to help fit, see the Palmer/Pletsch book **Fit for Real People**.*

NOTE: Don't be fooled into buying petite clothing if you are short. Short people often are the same waist length as a person who is 5' 6" tall, because all of their "shortness" is in their legs. Therefore, they wouldn't buy petite dresses that have a waistline. Also, as the size gets larger in petites, the garment gets longer.

* We are comparing to pattern measurements because they are standardized, whereas ready-to-wear sizing and grading varies a great deal from company to company.

Body Graph Worksheet

Name _____   Date _____

Body Size

Height   _____ Short (under 5′3″)   _____ Average (5′3″- 5′6″)   _____ Tall (over 5′6″)

Weight   _____ Slender   _____ Average   _____ Heavy

Body Shape (Silhouette – Use Body Graph)

Measure shoulder width (____″), waist (____″) and fullest hip (____″). Circle your predominant silhouette below:

Hourglass   Rectangle   Triangle   Inverted Triangle   Oval

Body Proportions (Use Body Graph and compare to "Ideal Proportions on previous page)

Head Length   _____ Short   _____ Average   _____ Long   (Average head fits between first two lines.)

Shoulders   For amount of slope, measure from shoulder dot straight up to line drawn out from neck base.
For width of shoulders, measure on shoulders from neck base dot out to shoulder dot.

_____ Even height   _____ Uneven   Left lower by _____ ″   Right lower by _____″

LEFT SHOULDER: _____ Sloping   _____ Average   _____ Square
_____ Narrow   _____ Average   _____ Broad

RIGHT SHOULDER: _____ Sloping   _____ Average   _____ Square
_____ Narrow   _____ Average   _____ Broad

NOTE: Shoulder width (neck base to shoulder) is 4¾″ in pattern size 10,
up to 5½″ in size 20. Shoulder slope is 1⅝″ in size 10, 2″ in size 20.

Draw line parallel to fold line.

*Measure **shoulder slope** from line to each shoulder dot.*

*Measure **shoulder width.***

NOTE: If one shoulder is sloping, that shoulder may also be longer.

Waist   _____ Small   _____ Average   _____ Thick
_____ Short   _____ Average   _____ Long
_____ Even height   _____ Uneven   Left lower by _____ ″   Right lower by _____″

Widest Hips   _____ Small   _____ Average   _____ Full   Left lower by _____ ″
_____ Even   _____ Uneven   Right lower by _____ ″
_____ Left fuller   _____ Right fuller   Center line to left full hip is _____″
Center line to right full hip is _____″

example: 8″   9″

Legs   _____ Short   _____ Average   _____ Long
UPPER LEGS: _____ Short   _____ Average   _____ Long
LOWER LEGS: _____ Short   _____ Average   _____ Long

Profile (Study your sideways profile in the mirror.)

Bust: _____ Small   _____ Average   _____ Full   _____ Low   _____ Average   _____ High

Tummy: _____ Flat   _____ Average   _____ Full

Derriere: _____ Flat   _____ Average   _____ Full

Chapter 3
Body Scale Connections

Women come in all heights, weights and body structures, which provides another opportunity to create visual connections. The goal is to find balance between your body scale and the details of your clothing and accessories. Think about the size you wear in panty hose, which is based on your height and weight proportions.

♦ An "A" panty hose woman is SMALL in scale, and looks best in petite prints, smaller collars, and daintier jewelry.

♦ A "B" or "C" panty hose woman is MEDIUM scale and balances with medium print motifs, garment details, and accessories. However, she can also move into the bolder end of small scale or the moderate end of large scale.

♦ A "D" panty hose woman is LARGE in scale. Her best look in garment details and accessories is medium to large.

♦ A "Q" panty hose gal has the physical presence to carry off striking, oversized jewelry. She would look silly wearing a delicate gold chain with a little gemstone pendant, for example. But her prints and garment details are best in medium to large scale. Small scale makes her look larger by contrast; extra-large scale makes her look larger by repetition.

Dana and Nicole are examples of larger and smaller scale. They differ in height and bone structure.

Nicole achieves balance with the two-strand necklace of small beads that would look insignificant on Dana. The necklace of larger stones balances with Dana's bolder scale, but it would swamp Nicole.

The dramatic gold earrings would overpower Nicole but Dana carries them off just fine. Nicole can wear the chandelier earrings successfully because, even though they are large overall, their small components and open structure give them a small-scale look.

These women probably wouldn't wear these earrings and necklaces at the same time. They donned them to illustrate our point.

Dana and Nicole

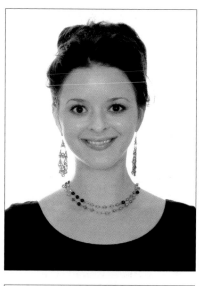

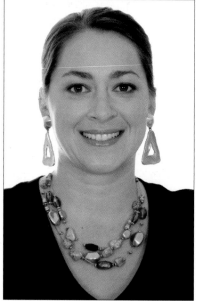

46

Even their scarf choices and the ways they wear them are influenced by body scale. The large square scarf, with its bold print of large bright flowers spread apart on a contrasting background, is in proportion to Dana's sturdy build. The smaller scarf and its proportionally small print motifs is in proportion to Nicole's diminutive stature.

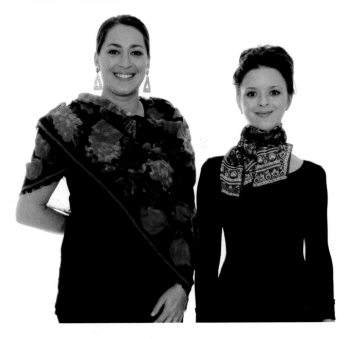

Modifying Factors

Of course panty-hose sizing is only one indicator of body scale. A woman's scale classification can be modified by factors other than her actual body size.

- **Coloring** – A woman with strongly contrasting coloring has a bold look that can allow her to successfully wear things slightly larger than her true physical scale. On the other hand, a woman with very pale or muted coloring has a gentler look that may connect with wardrobe details slightly more delicate than her true physical scale.

- **Personality** – An outspoken woman, a natural leader at home in the spotlight, often has the presence to scale up in her wardrobe choices. A more soft-spoken, behind-the-scenes gal may prefer to scale down slightly.

- **Personal style** – A woman with a dramatic, high-fashion approach to her wardrobe may enjoy scaling up a bit. One with a more casual, outdoorsy or romantic way of dressing may prefer to scale down slightly instead.

- **Bone Structure** – Hand and wrist size provide a good indicator of bone structure. More delicate wrists and small hands hint that a woman's scale would read smaller than her physical proportions would first suggest. Sturdier wrists and larger hands might move her scale in the opposite direction.

- **Athleticism** – A solid, athletic, muscular body can give the effect of a slightly scaled-up physical scale.

It is possible to manipulate scale somewhat to affect visual size. Which of the center circles looks larger? Both are the same size, but the one surrounded by smaller dots looks larger than the one surrounded by bigger dots.

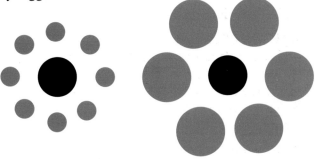

Using this concept carefully, you can minimize body size by adding slightly upscaled accessories or using print fabrics with slightly larger motifs. But carried too far this concept creates visual imbalance.

Below, rectangles A and C look larger due to the tiny dot pattern. The dots in D are so bold they look out of proportion with the rectangle. The mid-sized dots in B are a more balanced scale.

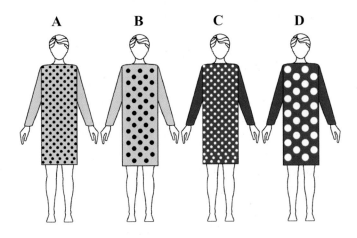

Chapter 4
Clothing Connections

Anyone, with any body type, can create the illusion of more balanced proportions through her choice of clothes. It's largely a matter of emphasizing assets and minimizing challenge areas through optical illusions. Five elements of design can help you achieve your figure goals:

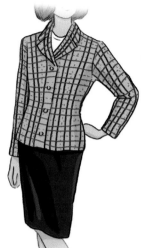

- ◆ **Texture** – Fuzzy, tweedy textures add visual bulk, while smooth surfaces minimize. Shiny, reflective surfaces enlarge; matte surfaces diminish.

- ◆ **Outside Line** – The silhouette or outline of a garment is most flattering when it echoes the outline of the wearer's body shape.

- ◆ **Proportion** – Unequal proportions in clothing are typically more flattering that equal proportions.

- ◆ **Inside Line** – The viewer's eye follows the design lines like seams, buttons, trims, pleats and lapels. Use these lines to draw attention where you want it. Vertical lines draw attention up and down, adding height and diminishing width. Horizontal lines add width, for better or worse.

- ◆ **Color** – Light, bright, warm colors attract attention and make the areas they cover seem larger. Darker, more subdued colors diminish.

Outside Lines

Many garments can be easily classified into the same five basic shapes we used to classify body shapes on page 46. Simply draw a mental outline around your garments. What shapes did you draw?

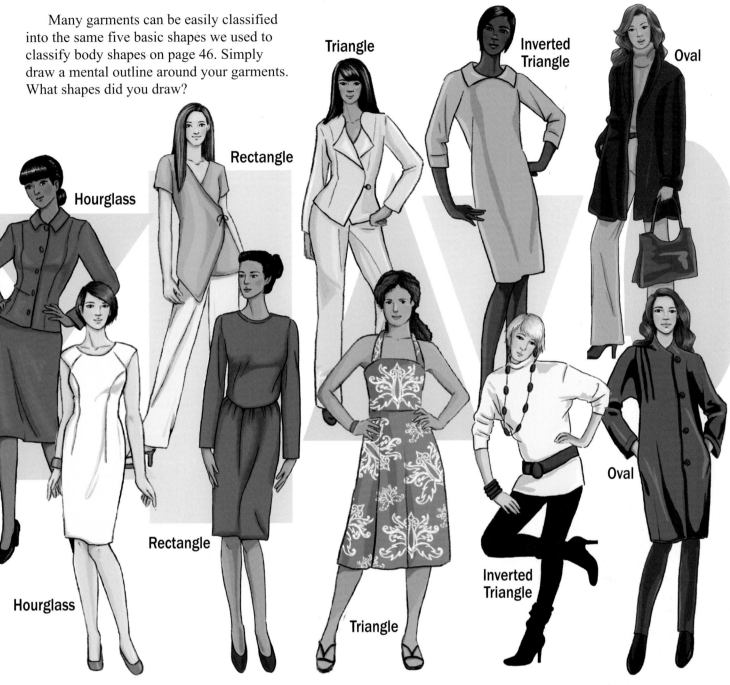

In general, the most pleasing outside lines are those that relate to your own body type. They are also the easiest styles to fit on you.

- **Hourglass bodies** look best in styles that follow or at least allude to their curved shapes. Darted waistlines, princess seams and body-skimming side seams create the desired shape.

- **Rectangle bodies** are flattered by straighter styles that skim right over their thicker waistline area.

- **Triangle bodies** need styles that enhance shoulders and fit easily over a fuller lower body without adding unwanted bulk.

- **Inverted triangle bodies** look best in styles that showcase their strong shoulder line and skim through the torso without adding hipline curve.

- **Ovals** need sleek styles with enough room through the waistline to avoid hugging the middle body.

You can use outside lines to make parts of your body look smaller by using optical illusion.

Which line looks longer? A or B? X or Y?

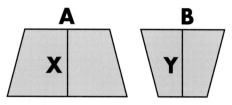

Although line A appears longer, it is actually identical to line B. Although Y looks longer, it actually matches X exactly.

The difference is the outside lines. When the outside lines angle outward the shape looks shorter and wider. When the outside lines angle inward, the shape appears taller and trimmer.

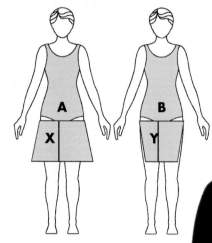

Now relate those abstract shapes to garments on a body like the skirt shown here. Which skirt makes the figure look taller and the hipline look more slender? This illusion makes a powerful argument in favor of gently tapered skirts and pants.

The same illusion illustrates the importance of creating a strong shoulder line with design details or subtle shoulder pads. When the silhouette tapers inward from shoulder to waist, the entire body looks taller and more slender. But when the lines from shoulder to waist taper outward, the body looks shorter and the waist looks fuller.

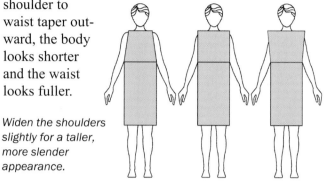

Widen the shoulders slightly for a taller, more slender appearance.

The shoulder line is one of the most critical points of design. Every body type is enhanced by strongly defined shoulders, though few of us have them naturally. Just look at supermodels and the grace with which clothes hang from their super shoulders.

Regardless of fashion trends, most women gain the illusion of a better balanced body when they add subtle shoulder padding. Removable foam pads can be moved from one garment to another, easily adding this figure-flattering detail to virtually every unstructured top in your wardrobe.

A bit of shoulder enhancement and gently tapering the slim skirt create a subtle but significant change in Victoria's figure balance.

50

Inside Lines

Inside lines move the viewer's eye up, down or across your body. They include details like:

- ♦ Collars and lapels
- ♦ Detail seams like princess lines and yokes
- ♦ Pleats, gathers and tucks
- ♦ Plackets
- ♦ Rows of buttons
- ♦ Trims and embroidery
- ♦ Pocket details
- ♦ Contrast topstitching
- ♦ Color change points
- ♦ Belts and sashes
- ♦ Epaulets
- ♦ Pocket flaps ... and more.

Vertical lines lengthen and narrow a body area or an entire silhouette.

Horizontal lines widen the area where they are placed and can shorten a silhouette.

Curved lines add softness. A curve that is primarily vertical can lengthen; a curve placed horizontally can widen.

Diagonals camouflage by leading the eye indirectly across the body. The more nearly vertical its orientation, the more a diagonal elongates a look.

Inside lines can be bold or subtle. The harder you have to look to identify them, the less they will affect your appearance. A row of contrasting buttons has more visual impact than buttons that match the garment. Seams and details that stand out on a solid color garment may virtually disappear in a print one.

Notice the inside lines of the garments below. They fall into four categories:

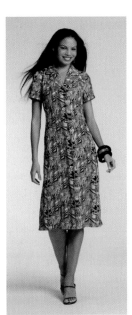
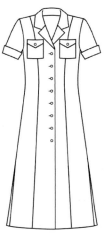

Inside lines disappear in the print.

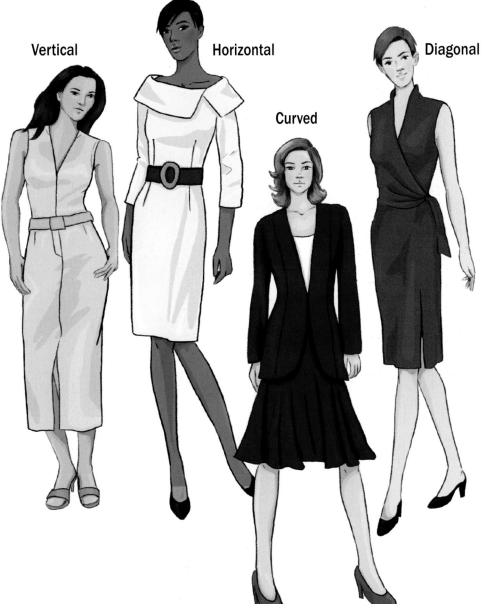

Vertical   **Horizontal**   **Diagonal**

Curved

Let's take a look at these four line types in action:

Verticals

An unbroken area looks wider than the same area divided into segments by a vertical line.

See how the figure on the left appears slimmer and taller? A center front seam, an inverted pleat, contrast placket, decorative zipper, or row of eye-catching buttons can create this flattering illusion.

A jacket worn open also creates a center vertical, but the effect is slimming ONLY if the jacket is open by choice, not if it is simply too snug to button.

A vertical line lengthens even more when the surrounding lines elongate it.

Which of these equal lines appears longer?

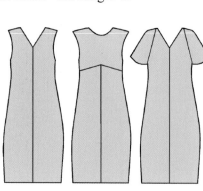

A V neckline combined with a center vertical is the ultimate in slimming design—so much that image consultants term this detail "the Magic Y."

In contrast, an empire seam or raglan sleeve detail can reduce the lengthening power of the center vertical.

But not all verticals are created equal. Which of these rectangles looks wider?

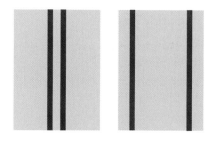

Two verticals placed near the center of the figure draw attention lengthwise and slenderize.

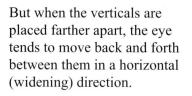

But when the verticals are placed farther apart, the eye tends to move back and forth between them in a horizontal (widening) direction.

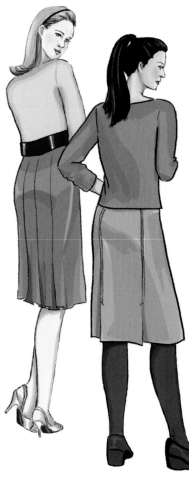

A series of many verticals (like stripes or pleats in a skirt) is more slenderizing if they are spaced more closely together.

NOTE: Widening isn't necessarily a bad thing. If applied to the upper body, for example, this detail could be effective to increase upper body size and balance fuller hips.

Horizontals

An unbroken area looks narrower than an equal area divided by a horizontal line.

But not all horizontals are created equal. Because a horizontal detail tends to hold attention, use one at a place you want to emphasize or enlarge.

For example, a contrast shoulder yoke, a wide collar, or pocket flaps can anchor attention on your upper body.

A flounced skirt hem calls attention to trim legs and away from a heavier torso.

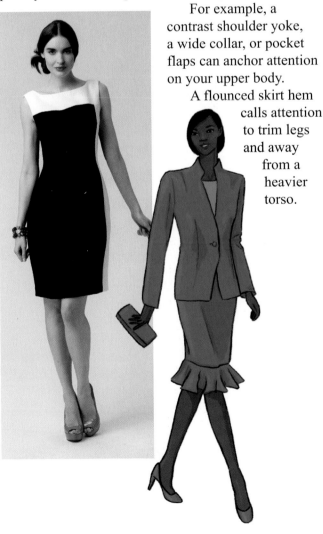

Two horizontals used together—like the yoke and waistband of a jean jacket—have more impact than a single one. The pocket flaps further emphasize the horizontal effect.

But a series of narrow, evenly spaced horizontals can actually draw the eye in an upward direction, like climbing a ladder. The blue and white stripes in the top below are an example.

Many women avoid horizontal stripes at all cost, afraid they'll be widening. But that isn't necessarily accurate. Big, bold rugby stripes in strongly contrasting colors do indeed widen; use them only on areas you want to increase for visual balance. Wearing a bold striped top can visually enlarge your upper body to balance fuller hips, for example.

But narrower stripes or variegated ones can actually lead the eye vertically as it "climbs the ladder" from one stripe to the next—go figure! And stripes with very little color contrast have about the same effect as a solid color—no horizontal direction at all.

Horizontals placed high or low on the body can slenderize the overall look compared with a horizontal that divides the figure evenly. The longer the eye moves up or down before meeting the horizontal, the taller and slimmer the figure will look.

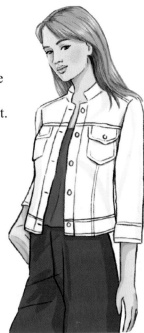

Narrow, evenly spaced horizontal stripes can draw the eye up just like climbing a ladder.

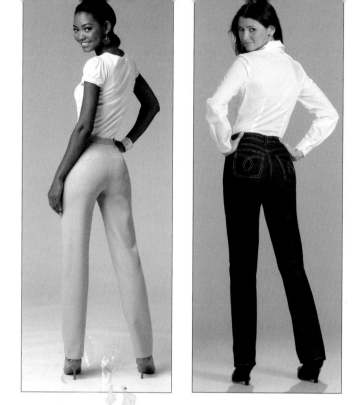

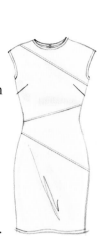

Diagonals

Diagonal lines can be very flattering because they divert attention past bust, waist or hips without stopping. The nearer a diagonal is to a vertical direction (far right), the greater the slenderizing impact.

Plaid fabrics are made up of vertical and horizontal lines. But cut on the bias they become diagonals and are much more figure-friendly.

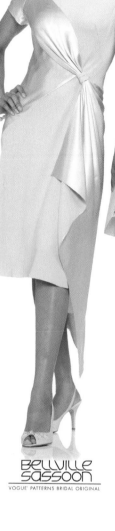

With these ideas about horizontals in mind, which is likely to be more flattering for the not quite ideal figure—tailored pants or jeans? The more defined the horizontal details are (contrast topstitching, for example), the stronger the widening effect becomes.

Understanding verticals and horizontals, you can improve the slimming potential of a double-breasted jacket:

♦ The widely spaced buttons (especially the nonfunctional upper pair) draw the eye from side to side, widening the torso.

♦ Simply snipping off the top buttons improves the look. Changing from contrast buttons to color-matched ones further minimize the horizontal impact.

♦ For an even more slimming effect, remove all but the lower functional button, creating an asymmetrical (diagonal) closure.

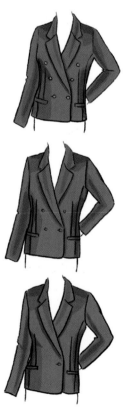

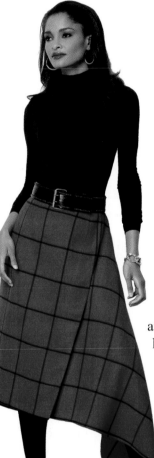

Diagonal hemlines also avoid a harsh, shortening horizontal break low on your body. They have the added advantage of showing more skirt length (at the longer points) and more leg (at the shorter points) so the lower body looks longer and leaner.

Triangles

The combination of diagonal lines and horizontals can create a visual triangle in clothing. When triangles occur, the eye tends to follow the horizontal line and see that body dimension as wider.

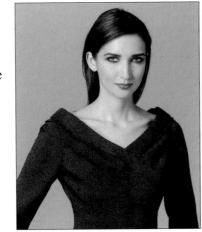

A wide V-neck creates a triangle that widens the shoulders.

A halter neckline forms a triangle that enhances the bust.

Curves

Curves are gentle, feminine lines, enhancing to many figures if used wisely.

They can add roundness to an awkward too-thin figure. The eye will follow a line until it ends or changes direction.

Therefore, a line curving upward will make the figure appear taller, while a line curving downward will visually shorten.

A curved hemline on a top or jacket avoids an abrupt horizontal at your hipline.

Simply shirring the side seams of a knit top can raise the hemline at the sides while leaving it longer at center front and back, creating the same flattering curved line.

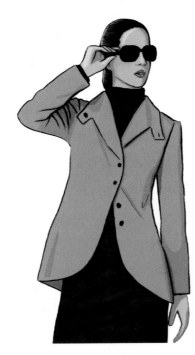

Converting/ Diverging Lines

Inside lines can also affect appearance when they come together (converge) or move apart (diverge). The area where the lines meet appears smaller; where they separate appears larger. The roll line and lapel edge of the jacket create lines that diverge to widen the shoulder area and converge at the tie closure, visually narrowing the waist.

The tucks radiating from the dress's neckline add visual fullness to the bust. A jacket that gaps open over full hips would be an unflattering example of this concept at work, making those hips look even fuller.

Hemlines

Hemlines are important horizontals that tend to stop the eye. Be sure they fall at flattering points on your body.

Fortunately fashion has moved away from rigidly dictated lengths. When it comes to hemlines, personal flattery trumps designer dictates every time. Remember, the fuller the pant or skirt style, the longer it needs to be to avoid a boxy look. A longer-than-wide proportion is nearly always more slimming.

Though hem preferences may vary, often one or two lengths are noticeably more flattering than others.

To determine the flattering skirt lengths for you:

♦ Stand in front of a full-length mirror in underwear and your favorite shoes. Hold a large scarf or length of fabric in front of you, draped to the floor.

♦ Raise and lower the fabric and notice how your legs look as the "hem" moves up and down.

♦ Find the narrow area just above your knee. That is the best short length for those whose knees can stand up to the exposure.

♦ Identify another narrow area barely below the knee, a flattering length for classic skirts.

♦ Find a third flattering length below the fullest part of your calf for longer and/or fuller styles. You probably won't wear a daytime skirt longer than this, except for resortwear.

♦ Ankle length is flattering for formalwear if your ankles are shapely and attractive.

♦ Floor length—just covering the shoe—is the universal length for formal occasions.

Notice that shorter women can wear the same variety of styles that flatter other women, since the decisions are based on positions along her leg length, not a specific length in inches.

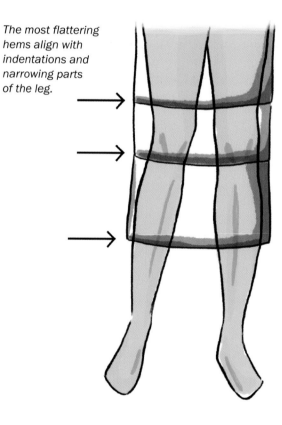

The most flattering hems align with indentations and narrowing parts of the leg.

Jacket Hems

Avoid a jacket hemmed to the fullest part of your hip, unless you need to look wider in that area.

♦ **Short jackets** generally work best paired with a skirt or perfectly fitted pant in a matching or receding color. They are most flattering on curved bodies (hourglass or triangle) and should have shaped side seams. They offer an easy fit for triangles, since they don't have to fit the hip area at all.

♦ **A hem just above the full hip** point works well on shorter women and those with balanced hips and shoulders.

♦ **Just below the full hip** is a versatile length to wear with both skirt and pants.

♦ **A hemline well below the hip** offers maximum coverage, but is very challenging to fit over a triangle figure. This length is usually better on taller women than on short ones. It works over pants or slim skirts, but not fuller styles, and is most flattering on straighter bodies (rectangles and inverted triangles).

Attention goes to any point where color changes abruptly from dark to light or dark to bright. An abrupt color change maximizes the horizontal line of the typical jacket hem, while a more subtle color change minimizes it. In an all-one-color suit, the jacket's hemline nearly disappears.

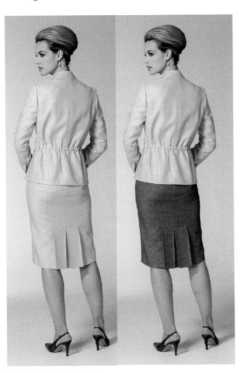

Pant Hems

The longer the pant leg, the longer your legs will look, provided the hem isn't dragging the ground. Heel height drastically affects pant length, of course, so always determine the hem with the shoes you intend to wear. Walk around in the garment for a minute or two, so the pants settle into their true position on your body.

♦ Straight-leg pants can break slightly over the shoe in front and angle down slightly in back to cover the point where the low heel meets the body of the shoe. For higher heels, bring the hem within about ¾" of the floor.

♦ Narrower legs have to be hemmed shorter, since they can't fit down over the top of the foot.

♦ Fuller legs can be hemmed nearly to the floor.

♦ Cuffed pants should be hemmed as long as possible, since the cuff itself forms a visually shortening horizontal detail. Most short women prefer to avoid cuffed pants entirely.

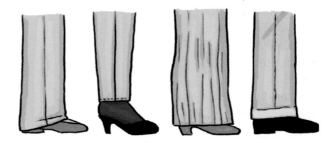

You can elongate the look of any pant hemline by the choice of shoes and hosiery. With a straight or fuller pant, avoid any visible skin and maintain color continuity by choosing a high vamp shoe that meets the hemline, or bridging the gap with dark trouser socks or tights. Pair casual skinny pants with short boots in a similar color or color value.

With a dressier narrow pant, you can't readily create color continuity because of the shorter hem. So try taking the opposite approach and reveal the maximum skin by choosing open toe, sling back or backless shoe styles.

Clothing Proportion

The relative proportion of color or design elements can make or break a look. A balanced 50:50 ratio is usually dull and uninspiring.

Unbalanced proportions are more pleasing to the eye. For example, pair a short jacket with a longer skirt or trousers. A longer jacket works best over a short skirt, not a mid-calf one. The ideal is to create a 3:5 ratio—the so-called Golden Mean. But a simpler 1:2 ratio is almost equally effective. In evaluating proportion in an ensemble, be aware that components other than the actual garments may need to be considered. For example, black tights appear as an extension of a black skirt. Dark brown hair extends the visual area of a dark brown jacket.

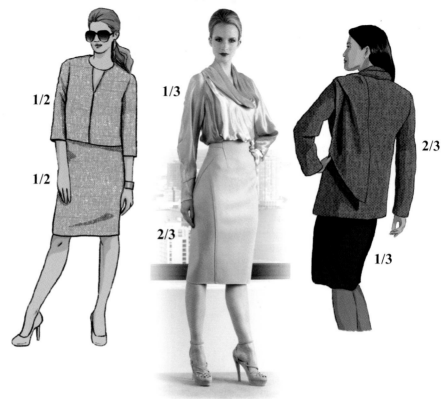

Texture

The look and feel of various fabrics can create proportional illusions too. Very textural, crisp, or shiny fabrics can increase visual bulk. Smooth, soft, matte fabrics tend to minimize.

Texture	Effect	Fabric Examples
Very soft and clingy	Follow body curves closely; too revealing for many figures	Single knits, silk jersey, chiffon, crepe de chine, charmeuse
Soft and drapable	Fall softy over curves; slimming in soft styles	Challis, georgette, lightweight gabardine, tissue faille, wool jersey, interlock knit, slinky knit
Moderately crisp	Hold garment shape away from body; flatter most because they don't cling	Dress linen, brushed denim, chino, gabardine, flannel, ponte knit
Very crisp	Stand away from body and enlarge figure	Linen suiting, heavier pique, heavy denim, satin, taffeta
Bulky, coarse, fuzzy	Enlarge the figure, can overpower a petite frame	Tweeds, thick sweater knits, velour, wide-wale corduroy
Smooth	Flattering to most figures	Gabardine, chino, ponte knit, challis, broadcloth
Shiny	Reflect light and increase body size	Satin, charmeuse, metallic
Dull, matte	Absorb light and minimize body size	Matte jersey, flannel, ponte knit, gabardine, interlock knit, crepe.

Clothing Connection to Silhouette

Hourglass Summary

An hourglass woman looks best in styles that repeat, or at least allude to, her curved shape and defined waist.

Her best jackets, shirts and dresses are shaped with darts, waistline tucks or princess seams. Ideal sweaters and knit tops are either shaped from the side seams or made from ribbed fabrics that shape to her body. Best skirts and pants rest at or just below her natural waistline rather than exaggeratedly low on her hips.

She generally looks best with tops tucked in and wears belts well, provided they aren't too wide for her torso length. Belting over a straighter shirt or jacket, however, usually creates a bulky, unflattering look.

Because of the defined fit through the waist, an hourglass needs to be careful that the waist-to-shoulder length of a shaped dress, shirt or jacket matches the length of her own body to avoid excess fabric forming horizontal wrinkles. A short-waisted hourglass may find her best fit in petite sizing even if she is taller than the traditional 5'4" cutoff for petites.

Although her hips and shoulders are balanced, most hourglasses still benefit from the subtle enhancement of small shoulder pads to slim the entire silhouette.

If an hourglass develops a bit of tummy fullness, she can eliminate front shaping in her tops, but retain the curved side seams and back darts or shaped seams to define her waistline.

Rectangle Summary

A rectangle looks best in straight or semifitted styles that enhance her more angular shape. Shaped dress styles will typically be too snug through the waist and create unflattering horizontal wrinkles. Shaped jackets will spread open at the waistline, pushing the lower edge into an awkward ruffle over the hips. However, garments shaped just below the bustline typically emphasize a narrow area of a rectangular body, simultaneously creating a flattering 1:2 proportion.

Longer jackets—from fingertip to duster length—are ideal for rectangles. Short styles call unwanted focus to the waist. The straighter blouses, tunics and jackets that suit a rectangular body retain a feminine mood when sewn in softer fabrics. Shaped shirttail hemlines or slits in the side seams add motion and softness.

Ready-to-wear pants or skirts with a traditional waistband are difficult to fit since a rectangle's waist is proportionally larger compared with her hips. Low-rise pants and styles with a waistline facing or drawstring all achieve an easier fit on rectangles.

Rectangles generally prefer shirts and sweaters worn out over the waistline of a skirt or pants.

Although rectangles often avoid belts because they don't want to call attention to their waistline, they can wear two styles of belts effectively:

- A narrow belt, color-matched to the garment and with an eye-catching buckle, visually narrows the waist by pulling attention to the center. This effect is even stronger when the outfit is topped with an open jacket. See page 114 for examples.

- A low-slung belt or chain belt worn asymmetrically creates the illusion of waistline curve. See page 115.

Diagonals are especially effective lines for rectangles, with their softening effect and ability to imply curves.

Triangle Summary

A triangle needs to balance her body shape by calling attention to her upper body, visually minimizing hips and maintaining the waistline definition of her curvy silhouette.

Triangles frequently make the mistake of trying to cover up hips with fuller pants and skirts and longer jackets. In fact, slimmer skirts and pants minimize lower body fullness. The secret is to purchase the garment to fit her hips and have the waistline taken in. Tapering the side seams furthers the slenderizing effect (see page 194). And keeping the bottom garments in darker, duller fabrics directs the visual attention to the trimmer upper body. Dresses and tunics with fullness designed to accommodate larger hips need to be made in softer fabrics to keep from adding visual pounds.

If a jacket is made in a brighter color, more interesting fabric pattern or texture, and with eye-catching details, it commands all the visual attention, allowing those hips to virtually disappear.

A jacket, shirt or top with a curved hemline—lower at center front, higher at the side seams—also avoids having to fit the hips.

61

Tucking a shirt or sweater into the bottom garment also moves the color break away from the hips, to the trimmer waistline, simultaneously elongating the lower body for a slimmer appearance overall.

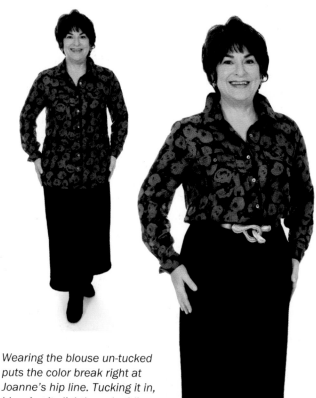

Wearing the blouse un-tucked puts the color break right at Joanne's hip line. Tucking it in, blousing it slightly and adding subtle shoulder shapers keep the attention at her upper body and waistline. Exposing the full length of the skirt makes her lower body look longer and slimmer.

Triangles always gain a more balanced look by adding medium-size shoulder shapers to balance upper body width to their fuller hips.

Tops designed to cover the hips have two disadvantages for a triangle figure:

♦ They place a horizontal hemline at the widest part of the body.

♦ They either fit the shoulder area and are a size or two too small through the hips, or they fit the hips and hang off the shoulders.

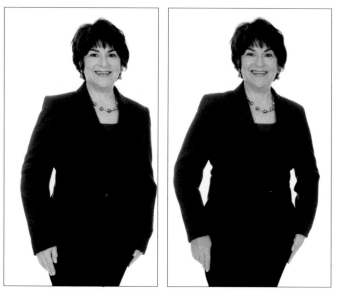

The jacket on the left fits Joanne's hips but is too large in the shoulder area. The one on the right fits her shoulders beautifully but pulls across her triangle body's larger hips.

Although it is possible to have the shoulder area taken in to fit correctly, that alteration is time-consuming and quite costly.

A surprisingly effective alternative is a shaped, above-hip-length jacket that sidesteps those fitting issues.

Inverted Triangle Summary

An inverted triangle needs to balance her proportions by minimizing her upper body and emphasizing her trim lower body.

Sleek shirt and jacket shapes, receding colors, smooth textures, and vertical design lines slim her upper body. Wearing a jacket open lets its front edge expose a vertical strip of the blouse color underneath.

Stronger colors, interesting patterns, and eye-catching design details in skirts and pants all draw attention to her slim hips and shapely legs.

At ideal weight, an inverted triangle can wear nearly any style successfully. In fact, almost all supermodels have this body type.

Fit can be a challenge. Her typical broad shoulders and full bust require a larger size in shirts and jackets, leaving extra fullness through the hip area that demands alteration.

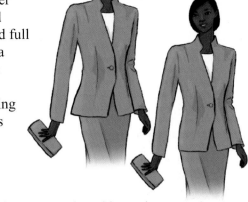

alter jacket at hips

Skirts and pants, purchased by waist measurement, typically need to be taken in through the hips. Low-rise pants and styles with a waistline facing or drawstring all achieve an easier fit on an inverted triangle.

This figure is also flattered by a low-slung belt, worn asymmetrically. This detail elongates her torso, making space for her full bust and avoiding a boxy look.

With maturity or weight gain, an inverted triangle can become thick through the middle body, making a more relaxed fit a better choice. Like the rectangle, an inverted triangle usually prefers to wear her tops untucked, skimming her waist area. She will also avoid jackets that end at her waistline.

Oval Summary

The goal for an oval is to strengthen her shoulder line to balance middle body fullness, while skimming through her waist area and creating attention up around her face.

Straight styles, without darts or princess seams to shape the waist, work best for this figure. Vertical design details—especially at the center front—give a longer, leaner look to her body.

A long jacket or vest, worn open, creates a visually dominant vertical. And a substantial shoulder pad gives lift and definition to the entire silhouette.

Tops generally look better worn out rather than tucked in. Jackets from fingertip to duster length are the most flattering. Ovals often find that sleeves are too full and need to be tapered to avoid adding visual bulk through the middle of the body.

Pants and skirts with elastic waist treatments give the oval figure the most dependable fit. The elastic finish isn't bulky because it stretches smooth to accommodate this fuller body area. Bottoms purchased for her relatively larger waist measurement may need to have the side seams taken in to avoid the sloppy look of excess fabric.

Details close to the face draw attention away from tummy fullness. A cowl neckline, contrast collar, eye-catching necklace (ending well above the bust), or bold earrings can all serve the purpose.

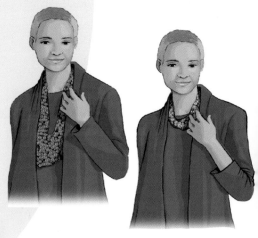

Wear accessories close to the face, like the necklace on the right, to bring attention up, away from the fuller part of the body.

The Inside Story

Each of the five body types can benefit from some of the newer developments in shaping undergarments. An outer garment can look only as good as the supporting under layers. Lumps and bumps can undermine the look of the loveliest dress. And a sagging bustline adds pounds and years to any woman's figure. See Chapter 13 for detailed information about conventional and shaping undergarments.

Double-Check These Image Details

When you've made the effort to choose the most flattering styles for your body type, you don't want any small details to undermine your look. Watch out for these subtle, and not-so-subtle, image saboteurs.

Problem	Solution
Rundown shoes	Work with a good shoe repair shop, use felt markers to touch up scuffs and scratches, put a piece of soft carpeting under your feet when you drive.
Nylons with runs	Keep a spare pair in your car's glove compartment or your desk drawer.
Underarm stains	Prevent them with dress shields or by trying a new deodorant; remove them from washable garments with a paste of baking soda and water.
Lint or dandruff	Keep a small lint brush or roller in your car or desk. In a pinch, wrap tape around your hand, sticky side out.
Missing buttons, snaps, hooks	If you can't repair them yourself, most dry cleaners offer this service.
Slipping bra straps	Notions departments sell tiny strap holders you can sew into the shoulder seam of any blouse. Or try the plastic clips that secure the straps to one another at center back.
Static cling	Use a commercial release spray, or rub a dryer sheet or just your own dampened hands over your body under the garment.
Visible underwear lines	Substitute or add panty hose to smooth panty lines; layer a smoothing spandex camisole over your bra. Try the vanishing-edge technology used in some panties.
Linings hanging too long	You or your dry cleaner can shorten the under layer.
Too-short coat over longer skirt	Buy coats extra-long with this issue in mind; they are warmer that way too.
Too-tight pants, skirts	If body-shaping undergarments won't solve the problem, either alter the garment or retire it.
Blouses gapping at the bust line	Try a minimizer bra; secure the garment edges with a double-stick garment tape like Flash Tape.
Sweater with pilling	Carefully remove the pills with a defuzz gadget or simple razor.
Snagged garment	Use a snag repair tool (found at sewing stores) to pull the snag to the back side of the fabric.
Faded garment	Consider dyeing it back to its original color—especially effective for washable black, brown or navy items.
Unkempt or outdated hairstyle	Work with a top stylist to find the right style for you, even if you have to use a more affordable salon for upkeep; master tools like Velcro rollers and flat irons to refresh your style quickly.
Roots, or technically, "regrowth"	Touch-ups can be expensive, so consider highlights or lowlights instead of overall color.
Rough cuticles	Push cuticles back with a towel after your shower; condition with a cuticle cream (or even lip balm) before bed.
Chipped polish	New quick-dry polishes and strong topcoats make manicures quick and long-lasting. Touch up polish in your car before you hit the road, so you have drive time for it to dry thoroughly.

Chapter 5
Make the Most of Your Body

Here are specific guidelines for applying the concepts of color, silhouette and style details to minimize common figure challenge areas.

Of course, the same characteristic that one woman considers her challenge may be another woman's favorite feature.

To Look Taller...

DO:

♦ If you are under 5' 3" consider shopping in the petite department, where the clothes are scaled to end at the same point on your shorter figure that regular size would end on a taller gal. (See page 44.)

♦ Create a longer line with vertical design features like front plackets, V necklines, narrow jacket lapels, jackets worn open, creased pant legs.

♦ Wear similar color values head to toe to create an unbroken lengthwise flow.

♦ Color-blend shoes and hosiery to avoid a distracting color break at the ankle. When possible, blend both to the color of your skirt or pant.

♦ Choose narrow, body-skimming silhouettes. Wear fuller styles only in soft fabrics that fall close to the body.

♦ Choose shoes with at least a 1" heel, even in casual styles. With a skirt, choose a low-vamp style to expose more leg length.

DON'T:

♦ Create widening horizontal lines with color contrast between top and bottom garments.

♦ Use horizontal details like hip yokes, trouser cuffs, bold pocket flaps, contrasting belts, and border-print hemlines.

To Look Shorter...

DO:

♦ Create horizontal emphasis with hip yokes, pocket flaps, trouser cuffs, wider lapels, bold belts, and horizontal stripes.

♦ Select contrasting colors for top and bottom garments.

♦ Keep garment details and accessories medium to bold in scale.

♦ Choose fuller styles like capes, swing jackets, and flared skirts.

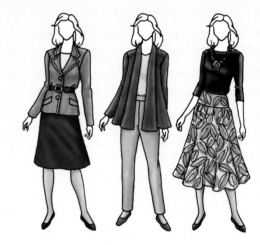

DON'T:

♦ Choose styles with too many vertical design lines.

♦ Wear one color head to toe.

♦ Choose style details, print motifs, or accessories that are too tiny for your body stature.

♦ Ever, ever wear pants or long sleeves that are too short.

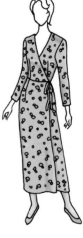

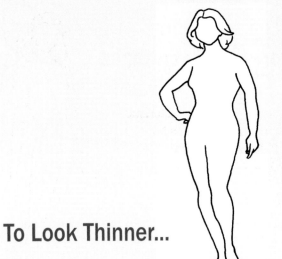

To Look Thinner...

DO:

- Use vertical design lines to lengthen and slenderize.

- Match or blend colors head to toe, including shoes and hosiery when feasible.

- Choose medium and darker colors, with brighter accents near the face to create a focal point.

- Strengthen your shoulder line with subtle shoulder padding to balance fullness lower on the body.

- Subtly taper slim skirts and pants for a narrower line.

- Choose fuller skirts only in longer lengths and soft, drapable fabrics.

- Try fluid wrap styles that skim over the body, forming graceful diagonal lines.

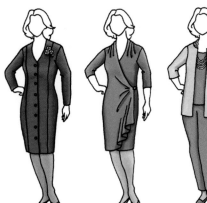

DON'T:

- Use widening horizontal lines lower than shoulder level.

- Wear anything too baggy— it adds bulk and looks sloppy.

- Wear anything too tight— it accentuates body fullness.

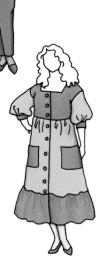

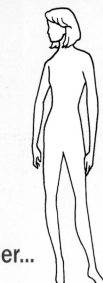

To Look Heavier...

DO:

- Choose horizontal details like yokes, wide belts, bold stripes, pocket flaps, trouser cuffs.

- Use gathers and soft fullness to create the illusion of added body bulk.

- Look for bulkier or highly textured fabrics like sweater knits, velour, tweeds, and wide-wale corduroy.

- Use multiple layers to create both fashion interest and body fullness.

- Color-contrast your top and bottom garments.

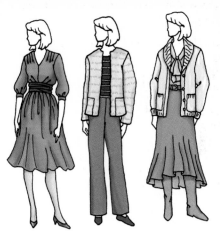

DON'T:

- Use too many vertical design lines.

- Choose clingy fabrics or body-hugging styles.

- Wear clothes too tight— it exposes thinness.

- Wear clothes too baggy— it accentuates the gap between your frame and the garment.

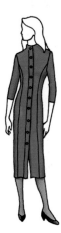

To Minimize Broad/ Square Shoulders...

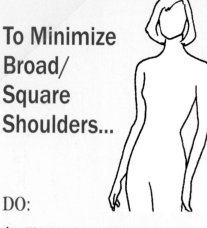

DO:

- Think twice—although it can be a fitting problem, this characteristic is usually a fashion asset.

- Choose raglan styles to create a sloping line.

- Create a vertical at the center of your torso with a V neckline, placket detail, narrow lapels of a jacket worn open.

- Create a center-body focal point with a center-tied scarf or a prominent neckline pin.

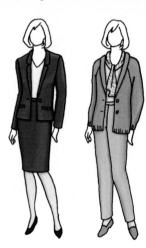

DON'T:

- Choose puffed sleeves or wide ruffled collars.

- Add shoulder details like yokes or epaulets.

To Broaden Narrow/ Sloping Shoulders...

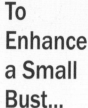

DO:

- Make a good pair of shoulder pads your fashion "best friend."

- Select details like yokes, epaulets, bateau necklines, set-in sleeves, or wide collars to maintain a horizontal shoulder emphasis.

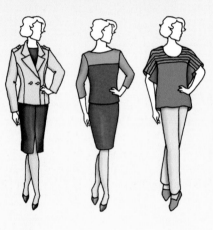

DON'T:

- Choose raglan-sleeve styles or halter tops.

- Select tent or swing styles that flare out from the shoulder line.

To Enhance a Small Bust...

DO:

- Invest in a maximizer bra—one that pushes breast tissue up and toward the center.

- Use layered tops to create visual fullness (sweater over shirt over turtleneck, for example).

- Wear bodices in lighter, brighter colors, with horizontal trims and breast pockets.

- Look for blouses with tucks, ruffles, soft draping, or blouson styling.

- Select short vests and bolero-style jackets.

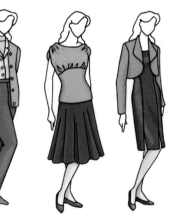

DON'T:

- Wear blouse styles that are tight-fitting or too low-cut.

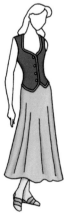

To Minimize a Full Bust...

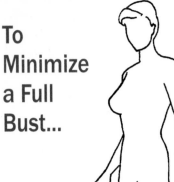

DO:

♦ Invest in a professionally fitted minimizer bra to distribute fullness side-to-side, reducing forward projection.

♦ Add subtle shoulder padding to balance bust fullness and eliminate downward drag lines in blouses and jackets.

♦ Shift focus upward with interesting necklines, scarves or jewelry. Or lower the focus with colorful skirt prints.

♦ Choose tapering jackets or over-blouses that end below full hip.

♦ Try blouson styles with just enough fabric to skim over body fullness.

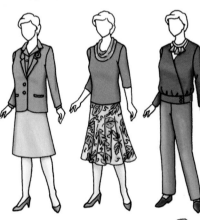

DON'T:

♦ Use horizontal bodice details like breast pockets or short sleeves with contrasting cuffs.

♦ Choose tight or clingy styles or wide belts or waistbands.

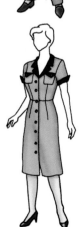

To Lengthen a Short-Waisted Body...

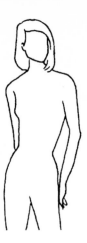

DO:

♦ Conceal the natural waist with dropped, raised or no-waistline styles.

♦ Choose jackets or blouses that cover or blouse over the waist.

♦ Try skirt and pant styles with waist facings instead of bands.

♦ Match belt color to bodice rather than bottoms.

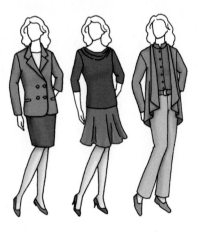

DON'T:

♦ Use horizontal bodice details (yokes, pockets) that visually shorten torso.

♦ Select full skirts that balloon out from the waist.

♦ Create a strong color break at your waist by tucking shirts or sweaters into your waistband.

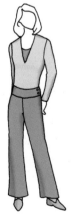

To Shorten a Long-Waisted Body...

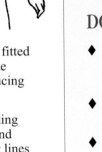

DO:

♦ Choose shorter jackets in bold, advancing colors, often with horizontal details in the lapels, pockets and trim.

♦ Use lengthening vertical details on the lower body for balance.

♦ Try raised-waistline skirt/pant styles, or wider waistbands.

♦ Color-match belts to trousers or skirt, not to bodice.

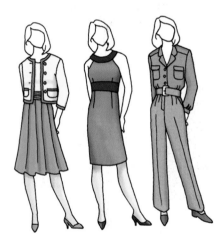

DON'T:

♦ Choose low-rise styles or faced waistlines instead of bands.

To Lengthen a Short Neck...

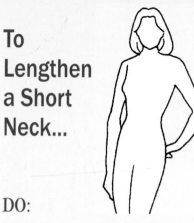

DO:

- Wear V necklines or open collars to elongate the neck.
- Keep earrings close to the ear, not dangling.
- Wear longer necklaces to expose more neckline area.
- Keep hairstyles short or upswept.

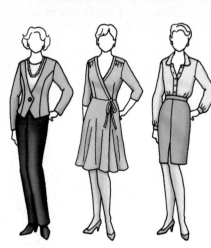

DON'T:

- Wear turtlenecks or other high necklines.
- Choose choker necklaces or tie scarves high on the neck.

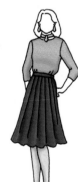

To Shorten a Long Neck...

DO:

- Realize that a long neck is often a fashion asset.
- Enjoy the ability to wear turtlenecks, choker necklaces, and other accessories close to the neck.
- Fill in the neckline area with longer, fuller hair.

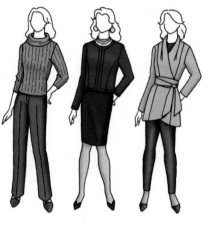

DON'T:

- Exaggerate the length with severe V necks in garments or jewelry.
- Choose earring styles that are very long and narrow.

To Lengthen or Slenderize Arms...

DO:

- Create the longest possible line from shoulder to wrist with tapered set-in sleeves or raglan styles.
- Use shoulder pads and details like epaulets to further enhance length.
- Keep cuffs moderate in size and color-matched to sleeve.

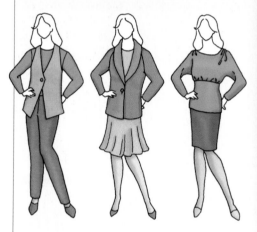

DON'T:

- Choose sleeves that are either too tight or too full.
- Wear short sleeves, especially ones with fitted cuffs.

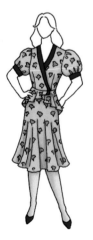

To Camouflage Long, Thin Arms...

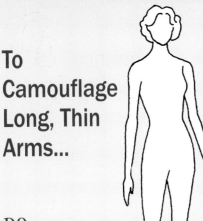

DO:

♦ Choose horizontal sleeve details like puffed, drop-shoulder, push-up, or short, cuffed sleeves.

♦ Find long sleeves with wide or contrasting cuffs.

♦ Be sure long sleeves are not too short; alter if necessary.

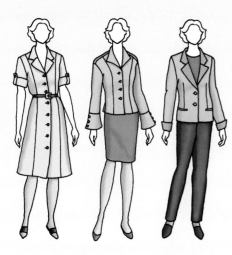

DON'T:

♦ Wear raglan-sleeve styling.

♦ Choose very tight sleeves.

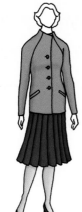

To Diminish a Prominent Tummy...

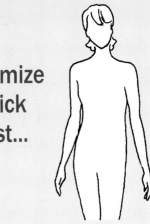

DO:

♦ Create a prominent shoulder line with shoulder pads, yokes, wide lapels, or horizontal collar styles.

♦ Wear styles that skim over the abdomen and taper at the hemline.

♦ Wear cardigans, swing jackets or shirt-jackets that conceal the abdomen. Pair them with tapered skirts or pants.

♦ Try longer blouson tops softly banded or tied below the tummy.

♦ Choose gently gathered skirts in soft fabrics.

♦ Draw attention upward with eye-catching scarves or neck-laces that end above bust level.

♦ Wear elastic-waist pants and skirts to fit your waist with minimum fullness in the hips and thighs.

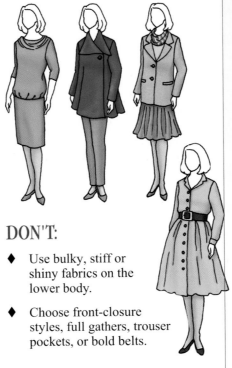

DON'T:

♦ Use bulky, stiff or shiny fabrics on the lower body.

♦ Choose front-closure styles, full gathers, trouser pockets, or bold belts.

To Minimize a Thick Waist...

DO:

♦ Keep belts and waistbands narrow and inconspicuous.

♦ Look for straight, body-skimming styles that obscure the waist, tapered at the hemline.

♦ Choose semifitted jackets with shoulder emphasis for balance. Wear them unbuttoned, for a slenderizing vertical band of blouse color underneath.

♦ Try a decorative belt buckle, worn under an unbuttoned jacket for a center-body focal point.

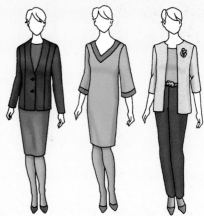

DON'T:

♦ Wear A-shapes in dresses or skirts.

♦ Wear wide or contrast-color belts.

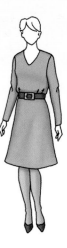

To Lengthen Short Legs...

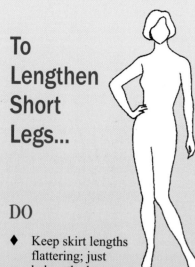

DO

- Keep skirt lengths flattering; just below the knee and just below the full calf are safe spots.
- Choose trouser styles with vertical details like fly-front closure, pleats, or creases.
- Look for skirts and pants with wider waistbands to elongate the look.
- Create an upward focus with bright tops and eye-catching jewelry.

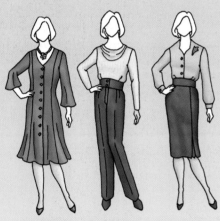

- Shop for skirts and pants in the petite department even if you need regular-size tops and jackets.

DON'T

- Wear pants/skirts with horizontal details (cuffs, yokes, patch pockets, border prints).

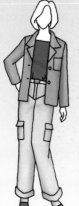

To Shorten Long Legs...

DO

- Wear sweaters, tunics or jackets that end at mid-thigh or lower.
- Match belt color to top garment, not skirt or pants.
- Choose pants with horizontal yokes, faced waistlines and cuffs.
- Hem fuller skirts to mid-calf length.
- Keep waistbands narrow or choose bottoms with a narrow binding or facing at the waist.

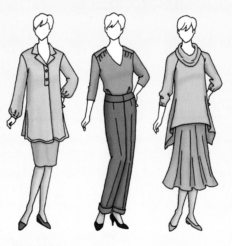

DON'T

- Tuck fitted blouses into high-rise waistlines.

To Enhance Narrow Hips/ Derriere...

DO

- Choose flared or gathered skirts in moderately crisp fabrics.
- Try jackets with peplums or swing styles to add hipline fullness.

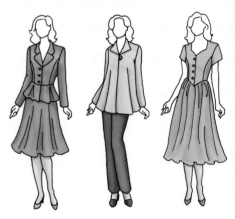

DON'T

- Wear pants or skirts with baggy fullness below the derriere. Alter if necessary for proper fit.

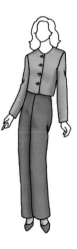

To Slenderize Heavy Hips/ Thighs/Derriere...

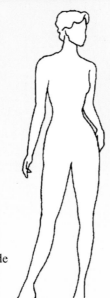

DO

- ◆ Broaden shoulders with shoulder pads, yokes, and wide collars to balance hips.

- ◆ Use brightly colored tops with eye-catching details tofocus attention on the upper body.

- ◆ Select dark-colored skirts or pants that skim over the hips and taper at the hemline for a narrower look.

- ◆ Look for skirts with center-front pleats or plackets to draw the eye toward the center of the figure.

- ◆ Choose jackets that end above or below the widest part of hips.

- ◆ Tuck in shirts and choose jackets that end between the waist and high hip.

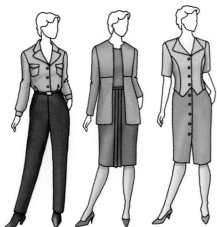

DON'T

- ◆ Position any eye-catching details at the hipline (yokes, pockets).

- ◆ Wear pants too tight, creating horizontal wrinkles. Buy to fit the hips and alter the waist.

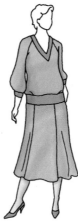

You don't have to be a perfect size 6 to dress with style and flair.

73

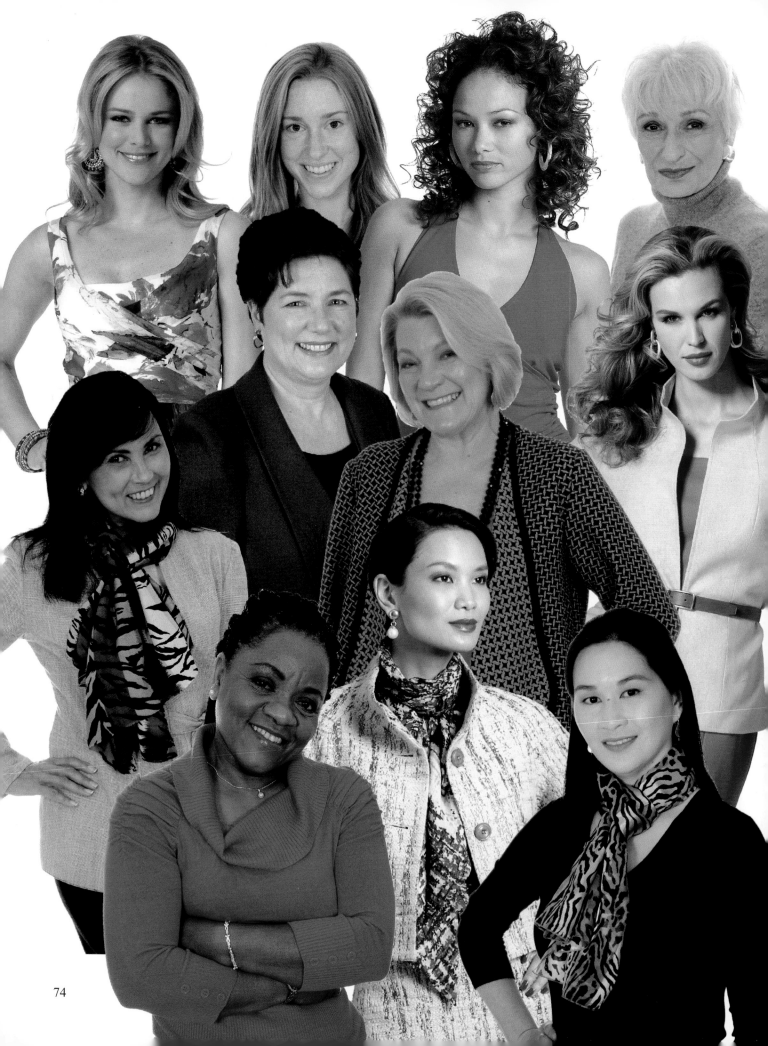

Chapter 6
Facial Connections

Because your face is such a prominent part of your appearance, it's especially important to create visual connections between its outline and its features and the items in your wardrobe.

Facial Shape Connection

Although some resources define a variety of facial shapes, the important variable is the height:width ratio. The presumably "ideal" oval shape is a ratio of about 5" wide to 7" long. You don't need to get out a tape measure—just look to see if your face from hairline to chin is about one and a half times its width at the jaw line. If it is, you can successfully wear most hairstyles, necklines, and jewelry shapes.

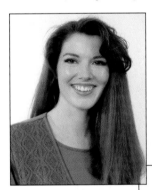

Wide

If your face is wide relative to its length, you can appear slimmer overall by using some simple techniques to make your face look longer and narrower:

- Push any bangs off your fore-head, sweeping them up and back for some subtle lift instead.

- Minimize the fullness at the sides of your hairstyle— perhaps by pushing the hair behind your ears.

- To expose more neck, tie scarves lower and wear open necklines and lower necklaces.

- Choose earrings that are longer than they are wide, though not necessarily long dangles.

- Style your eyebrows to emphasize an arch rather than a straighter horizontal shape.

- Apply your blush in a diagonal rather than horizontal direction.

Long

A slightly longer facial shape can be an asset, creating an automatic illusion of a trimmer body. But as the length proportion increases, the result can be an unfriendly or unwelcoming appearance.

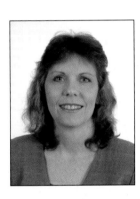

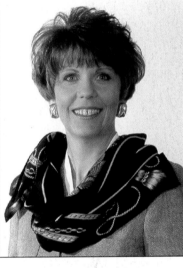

To soften a long facial shape:

- Add soft bangs to your hairstyle to cover a prominent forehead.

- Maximize fullness at the sides of your hairstyle, too. Shorter styles are usually more flattering for long faces.

- Wear higher necklines, or fill in lower ones with a scarf or choker necklace.

- Choose earrings that are a bit wider than they are long.

- Style your brows to flatten the arch, creating a more horizontal shape.

- Apply your blush in a horizontal rather than a diagonal direction.

Facial Structure Connection

Within the outline of your facial shape, your features have a structure of their own. Your mouth, eyes, nose, brows, and cheekbones can be described as being decidedly angular, decidedly curved, or somewhere in between. (Although some people tend to associate curved features with weight gain, that is not actually the case at all.) Envision the angles in faces like Cher or Sarah Jessica Parker, and then contrast them with the curved features of Rosie O'Donnell or Oprah.

Many writers advise wearing the opposite shapes to counteract your curves or angles. But we believe you'll see greater harmony when you repeat those characteristics instead. Remember, you're beautiful just the way you are.

Your degree of angle/curve defines your most enhancing shapes for garment details, print motifs and accessories.

Angular

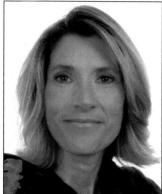

A woman with angular facial features will find harmony with geometric prints and plaids, square or rectangular earrings, squared pockets and jacket hems, peaked jacket lapels, boxy handbags, squared or pointed-toe shoes, and other angular details.

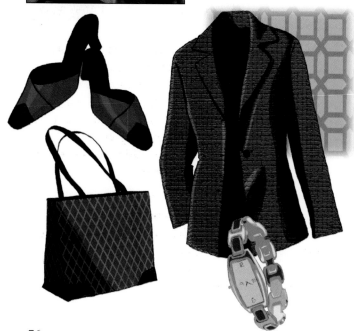

Curvy

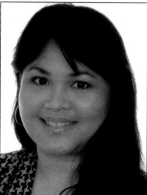

A woman with curved features will find rounded print motifs, circular earrings, curved pockets and jacket hems, shawl collars, softly curved handbags, and rounded-toe shoes more compatible.

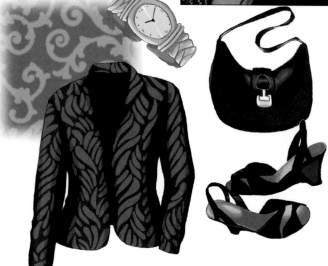

And In Between

Women with more mid-level features will be flattered by mid-level or blended design details:

♦ A jacket with traditional lapels, neither rounded nor as angular as the peaked styling.

♦ A square earring, but one that has curved dimension, rather like a little pillow.

♦ Shoes with an elongated but rounded toe shape.

♦ A plaid fabric, but in soft colors so the look of the right angles is softened.

Building a wardrobe that is consistent in its degree of angularity means all the components will have inherent compatibility with one another as well as with you. Mixing and matching becomes far easier when, for example, the shape of your belt buckle relates to the squares of your plaid jacket and the angles in your shoe shape.

Facial Scale Connections

Regardless of your overall body scale, your facial features have a scale of their own. The two may match or they may differ.

When you are choosing wardrobe details that will be worn near your face, they need to relate to the scale of your features. The model below has a sturdy, athletic frame but her facial features are small by comparison. Her ideal accessories are fairly bold scale to match her body scale, but are made up of many small components that relate to her facial scale.

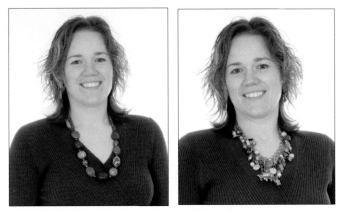

The bold beads balance with her body scale but overwhelm her smaller features. The charm necklace is bold overall, but the small individual charms relate to her facial scale.

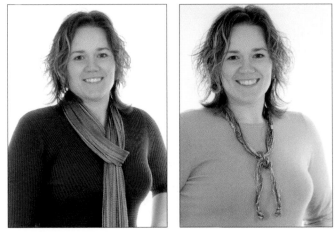

The narrow stripes in the scarf and the individual strands in the knotted necklace also give a lighter scale within an item of overall bolder dimensions.

Textural Connections

Your hair and face have texture, and you can repeat that texture for a beautiful effect.

♦ If your skin is smooth and uniform in color and your hair is sleek, you'll look best in fabric surfaces that appear smooth.

♦ Personal texture patterns like freckles, curly hair, or variegated hair color (natural or highlighted) balance best with equally textured fabrics. Many small prints also give the appearance of this level of texture.

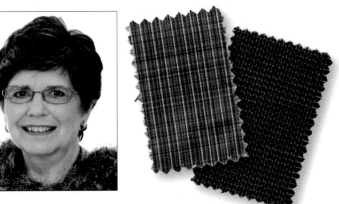

Tamara's curly hair and light freckles are coplimented by fabrics with textured surfaces or by small, dimensional prints that give the appearance of texture.

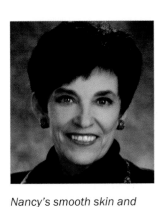

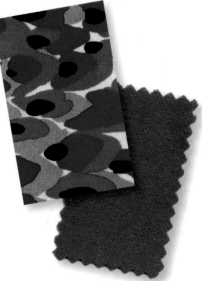

Nancy's smooth skin and straight, uniformly colored hair relate well to smooth surfaces and well-defined print motifs.

♦ A woman with extremely textural hair and skin might prefer to repeat that texture in her lower-body garments and wear a less-textured bodice to avoid a too-busy look. For a recent client with long kinky-curly red hair and lots of prominent freckles, we used this approach to give the viewer's eye a bit of rest while still echoing her textural pattern within the outfit.

♦ Even a textural characteristic that isn't your favorite still benefits from repetition. Fine lines and wrinkles, for example, look more pronounced when framed by very smooth surfaces, but appear less noticeable when surrounded by lightly textured ones.

Chapter 7
Lifestyle Connections

Your wardrobe needs not only to connect with your physical characteristics—it also needs to connect with your lifestyle.

Where do you go? What do you do? And what do you need to wear?

The answers to these questions change throughout a woman's life. Student … young professional … working parent … at-home mom … returning professional … retiree. All of our lives are a succession of roles.

And to complicate matters even more, we may wear a variety of hats during any one stage. It's important to have a wardrobe that meets ALL our lifestyle needs, or we can easily go astray.

♦ Many professional women have closets full of beautiful career wear, but dress like a "ragbag" in their leisure hours and struggle with what to wear for a casual social event.

♦ At-home moms may have plenty of casual clothes but nothing to wear for a special occasion.

Lifestyle Chart

	HOURS SPENT DAILY							Weekly Total
	Sun.	Mon.	Tues.	Wed.	Thur.	Fri.	Sat.	
Professional Time								
Full-time work								
Part-time work								
Volunteer work								
Family Time								
Mothering								
Cooking								
Shopping								
Other household activities								
Social Time								
Church								
Entertaining								
Entertainment (dining out, cultural activities)								
Recreation Time								
Sewing/Arts/Crafts								
Gardening								
Sports								
Relaxing/TV time								
Other								

Professional

professional

social

sports

family

Working Parent

professional

family

social

sports

Homemaker/ Mom

volunteer/ professional

family

social

sports

Take a look at your lifestyle using the chart below. Then calculate the percentage of time you spend in each category of activities. Create a pie graph to give you a visual image of your wardrobe needs.

The mix of clothing in your closet—your Wardrobe Pie—should align closely with your Lifestyle Pie.

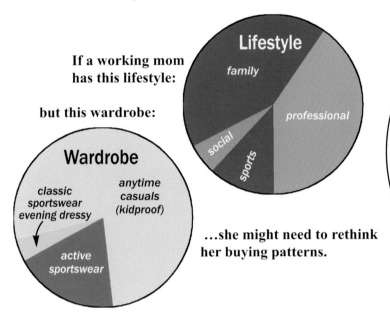

If a working mom has this lifestyle:

but this wardrobe:

...she might need to rethink her buying patterns.

Clothing categories should match their corresponding lifestyle categories:

- Career clothing in proportion to your working hours.
- Casual sportswear in proportion to your at-home time.
- Daytime dresses in proportion to church/social activities.
- After-five clothing in proportion to your evening occasions.
- Action wear in proportion to your fitness and sports time.

That balance needs to exist in terms of wardrobe VOLUME, not necessarily wardrobe BUDGET, since clothing in some categories (like career) can be considerably more expensive than in others (like casual sportswear). However, that doesn't mean an at-home mom should default to lots of cheap jeans and sweats instead of fewer, nicer pieces. It's important for your family to see you dressing well, even in casual clothes. And you'll feel more special too.

It's also important to have something to wear for any occasion that might arise. What could you find in your closet to wear to a daytime wedding? A charity gala? A funeral? You may not be able to fill all those categories at once, but make it a goal to be ready to dress for all of life's surprises.

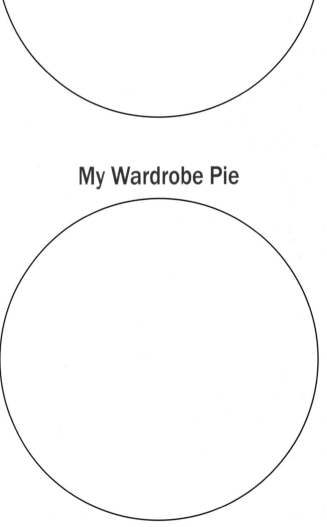

My Lifestyle Pie

My Wardrobe Pie

Career Connections

Back in the 1970s women sneaked into the work force disguised as men. Remember all the navy blue suits, white shirts, and red bow ties? Or maybe you've just read about them. A lot has changed since then! Women have earned their place in the business world and today our unique attributes aren't just accepted, they're prized.

That acceptance brings the flexibility to express our own style in a variety of career clothing, including business casual. It's important to analyze the impact of various business looks and be sure your appearance connects with the message you want to communicate.

Unfortunately, many women (and men too, of course) have taken the idea of business casual to extremes and sacrificed their credibility for the comfort of jeans, sweatshirts, and sneakers. Even in casual environments it makes sense to dress well. Career strategist Marilyn Moats Kennedy says, "I have never seen a job where it pays to look less than your best."

This chart outlines some of the messages women in various career fields might want to convey and the types of clothing that communicate them.

BUSINESS	Law, Banking, Finance, High-level Corporate	Insurance, Real Estate, Sales	Advertising, Art, Fashion, Writing, Entertainment
MESSAGES	Authoritative Conservative Competent	Trustworthy Approachable Knowledgeable	Creative Individual Contemporary
CLOTHES	skirt suits, pant suits, and tailored dresses, mostly neutral solid colors, high quality fabrics, classic styling, conservative accessories	softly tailored coordinates, sweater jackets, more color variety and patterned fabrics, fashion accessories	More individualized style accepted, even expected; less structured garments, bolder colors and patterns, unique accessories

Every component of an outfit can move the look along the scale from most formal/authoritative to most relaxed/creative. In general:

♦ Solid colors are more authoritative; patterned fabrics are more relaxed.

♦ Darker, more neutral colors are more authoritative; brighter or paler colors are more relaxed.

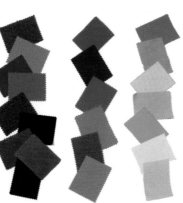

♦ Small geometric patterns in neutral or classic colors— whether woven or printed—are more authoritative; larger patterns in brighter colors usually feel more informal.

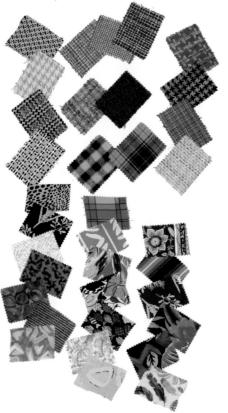

♦ Smooth-surface fabrics are more authoritative; very textural fabrics are usually more relaxed.

♦ Tailored jackets are more authoritative; unstructured jackets are more relaxed.

♦ Crisp fabrics are generally more authoritative; soft fabrics are more relaxed.

Understanding these guidelines makes it easier— even in relatively casual industries—to dress for the job you want rather than the job you have. Pay close attention to the appearance of role model women in the job levels above yours. You'll find ways to subtly make it easier for managers to "see" you in one of those roles too.

Even a relatively conservative business environment allows for some self-expression in a career wardrobe. Here is how a basic gray suit can be personalized for various women and their bodies, coloring, and personal styles.

Personalizing the Basic Gray Suit

Create a sportier feel with a ribbed sweater, natural leather belt, and gauze paisley scarf.

A silk dot blouse and pearl choker give the suit a classic look.

Soften and feminize the look with a blush draped shell and latticework necklace.

Working at Home

These days many women work from their homes, and face some special wardrobe challenges. Client meetings and presentations may require the traditional dress for their particular profession. And even home-office time requires a polished casual wardrobe. Dragging around in sloppy sweats or jeans undermines any feeling of professionalism and credibility. The information on capsule wardrobing, page 105 can help address these specialized needs.

Chapter 8

Personal Style Connections

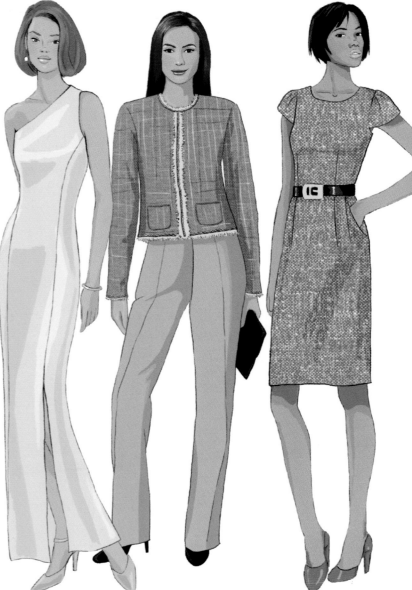

Dressing well is more than connecting your clothes and accessories to your physical attributes (or coloring, body shape, and facial characteristics). It's also about who you are and what you project as a person—your personal style.

Have you ever had an outfit that, every time you wore it, gave you the wonderful feeling of "This is just ME"? It undoubtedly was a reflection of your personal style—your inborn tendency to feel the most authentic in a particular way of putting yourself together.

Some experts believe a woman dresses a certain way because her lifestyle or her career demand it. But we feel that the same internal compass directs her simultaneously to a job, a life, and a look that are congruent expressions of her authentic self.

So who is this woman you want to dress? You need to know, so you can have that "It's just ME" experience all the time on purpose instead of once in a while by accident. Many women find themselves fitting easily into one of these five style categories: **Classic, Sporty/Natural, Dramatic, Romantic,** or **Artistic.**

Classic

The Classic woman is drawn to traditional, refined clothing and understated accessories. She isn't likely to jump on passing trends, preferring to invest in quality fabrics and timeless styles instead. Simple lines, balanced proportions, and symmetrical designs characterize her wardrobe.

She usually chooses solid color fabrics or small patterns like herringbone or houndstooth. In prints, she is likely to prefer paisleys or controlled geometrics over larger, bolder designs. She tends to avoid fabrics that are either bulky or clingy, opting instead for fine woolens, silks, and jersey.

Her jewelry choices are usually geometric shapes in elegant materials like pearls and semiprecious stones. Classic pumps and loafers fill her shoe closet and her handbag is probably a conservative size, relatively structured, and without bold pattern or excess embellishment.

Caution: A tailored Classic woman is sometimes so cautious about avoiding extremes that she ends up looking so safe and conservative—even boring. She may need to step just outside her natural comfort zone to spice up her look with a few interesting fashion touches, like the red shoes, above.

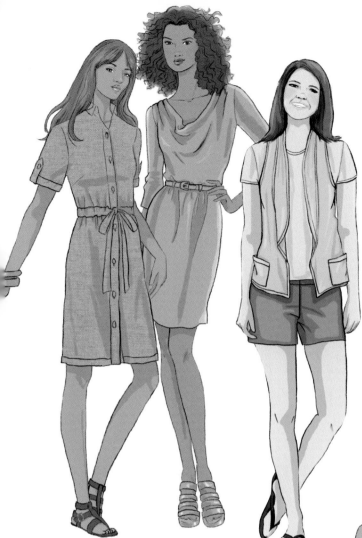

Sporty/Natural

A Sporty/Natural is an easygoing casual person who is not willing to suffer for the sake of fashion. Comfort and practicality are basic requirements for her wardrobe choices. Seasonal trends seldom get her interest.

She leans toward fabrics like denim, corduroy and tweeds, shirting plaids and stripes, T-shirt knits and cozy sweater knits. She is usually drawn to subtle colors rather than sweet pastels or bold brights.

Her jewelry choices are usually basic and durable—chunky leather belts, simple chain necklaces, basic stud earrings, a sporty watch. She chooses sturdy loafers or sneakers for casual wear and low-heeled pumps or wedges for dress. She probably carries a shoulder bag or backpack.

Caution: A Sporty/Natural can easily look under-dressed. She needs a good haircut, a few polished accessories, and good fit to avoid the risk of looking sloppy.

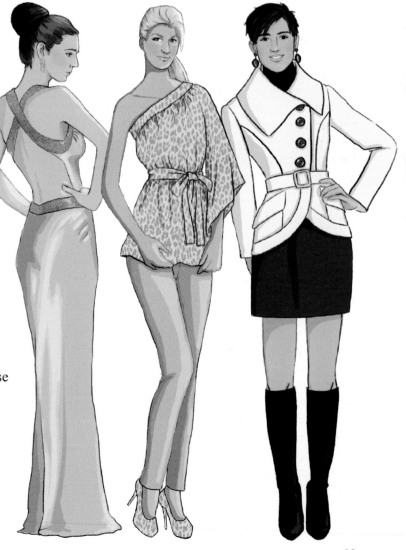

Dramatic

Typically a clotheshorse, the Dramatic loves to be seen in the latest styles. For her, comfort takes a backseat to fashion. Bold colors, oversized details, and asymmetrical design lines characterize her striking, head-turning look.

Her closet is typically full of solid colors—often worn in bold, unexpected combinations—and smooth fabrics like gabardine, satin, crepe, and jersey. Print choices run toward bold, oversized geometrics and abstracts.

Her jewelry pieces make bold statements, maybe large geometric pieces in shiny metal finishes or perhaps one-of-a-kind wearable art items. Her purse is probably oversized and makes a statement in style, texture or detail. Her closet is likely to be filled with interesting colored shoes and tall boots.

Caution: A high-fashion Dramatic can easily overdo her bold look and overpower or intimidate less fashion-forward acquaintances. She may need to consciously tone down her flamboyant look, especially if she works in a corporate environment.

Romantic

The Romantic has a soft, feminine appearance and generally prefers soft silhouettes, gentle colors, and rounded design details.

Her fabric choices are typically lightweight and drapable. Soft jerseys, silks, challis, crepe and voile appeal to her. These soft fabrics let her wear volume without creating excess bulk. In prints she is likely to prefer florals or other soft motifs. Details like lace and bows may show up in her clothes and accessories.

Femininity is the key to a Romantic's accessory choices. Smaller scale, softly colored pearls or gemstones, and curved shapes predominate. Bow and floral motifs, cameos and vintage-look pieces often appeal to women with a Romantic style. Her shoes are visually lightweight (think ballet flats or kitten heels) and handbags tend to be soft and relatively small.

Caution: This style type needs to be careful to avoid coming across fluffy or little-girlish, especially in business situations.

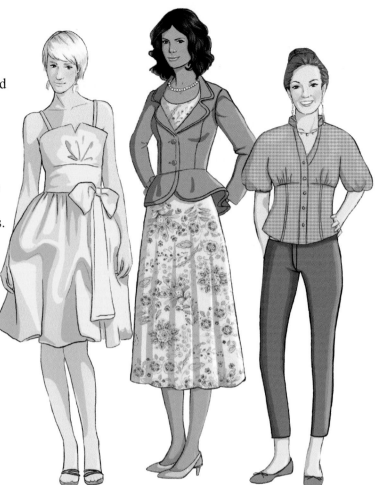

Artistic

The Artistic has her own highly creative and imaginative way of dressing—innovative and individualistic. She isn't overly influenced by either current trends or traditional "rules." Her aesthetic sense allows her to express her personality through attractive, though nontraditional wardrobe mixes.

Her fabric choices are infinitely varied, and often combined in unexpected mixes like lace with leather or brocade with denim. Home decorator and even industrial fabrics can find their way into her wardrobe.

Complex colors (not bright primary tones) and unconventional mixes contribute to her art-to-wear aesthetic. When she chooses prints they are likely to be equally unconventional, with motifs from art elements to birds and animals to vintage.

Eclectic is the best description for her accessories: kitschy, glitzy, handmade, vintage and other unusual styles of jewelry, shoes and handbags function as design elements to create her one-of-a-kind outfits.

Caution: This style type needs to avoid expressing a degree of nonconformity that makes her seem unapproachable or out of step with her social or business surroundings.

Clues to Your Personal Style

These categories are only a sampling of the range of personal styles. If you don't see yourself in one of them (or see yourself in all of them), don't worry. Rather than trying to force yourself into any preset category, we invite you to develop your own unique Personal Style Formula.

Find clues by pulling three or four favorite outfits or individual pieces out of your current closet—things you feel wonderful wearing and wouldn't dream of purging from your life. What adjectives could describe what your choices have in common, or describe the woman who would wear them all?

If your brain is stuck, scan the list below for words that describe your personality, your passions, your inner spirit … the traits that make you, YOU. They will probably apply to those special clothes, too. Of course our list is just to get you thinking. You can add any other words that feel right for you.

- ❏ adorable
- ❏ artistic
- ❏ bold
- ❏ classic
- ❏ classy
- ❏ cuddly
- ❏ dashing
- ❏ dazzling
- ❏ delicate
- ❏ dramatic
- ❏ dynamic
- ❏ earthy
- ❏ eclectic
- ❏ elegant
- ❏ energetic
- ❏ exotic
- ❏ fancy
- ❏ feminine
- ❏ flashy
- ❏ fragile
- ❏ funky
- ❏ genteel
- ❏ gentle
- ❏ glitzy
- ❏ graceful
- ❏ high-fashion
- ❏ ladylike
- ❏ mysterious
- ❏ natural
- ❏ offbeat
- ❏ old-fashioned
- ❏ outdoorsy
- ❏ polished
- ❏ romantic
- ❏ sophisticated
- ❏ sparkling
- ❏ sporty
- ❏ strong
- ❏ sturdy
- ❏ traditional
- ❏ unique
- ❏ whimsical
- ❏ zany

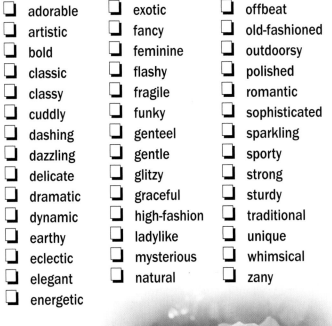

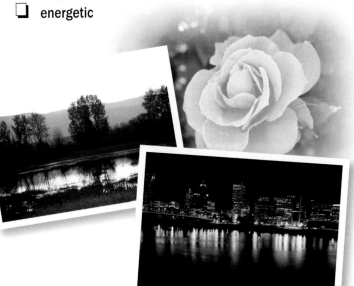

Start a Style File to Find Your Personal Style

Still struggling to define your personal style? Then try this exercise adapted from the book *Simple Abundance* by Sarah Ban Breathnach.

Flip through catalogs and magazines, snipping pictures of things that resonate for you. Clothes that make your heart sing. And images of other things too … scenes, homes, people … whatever speaks to your spirit. Don't censor your choices. Never mind that the jacket isn't your color, the dress wouldn't flatter your body type, or you don't have any place this week to

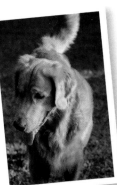

wear those cowboy boots. This exercise is all about feelings. Most people find that a theme develops fairly quickly.

- ◆ Lot of outdoor scenes. Earthy colors. Hearty food. SUVs. Golden retrievers.

- ◆ Roses. Chiffon. Lace. Babies. Candlelight dinners.

- ◆ City skylines. Urban sculpture. Art galleries. Contemporary furniture.

Which words from the list at the left characterize your picture collection? They very likely describe your style, too. The possibilities are infinitely variable. For example:

- ◆ The outdoorsy images might lead you to descriptive words like *earthy, sturdy, strong,* and *rustic.*

- ◆ Pictures of roses and candlelight could point to a style formula that includes words like *adorable, cuddly, delicate,* and *genteel.*

- ◆ The urban architecture could elicit descriptions like *artistic, bold, high-fashion,* and *sophisticated.*

Still stuck? Try scanning the list once more and crossing off the words that don't resonate for you at all. Some women find that approach leads them more easily to a personal style formula by process of elimination.

Chapter 9
Closet Connections

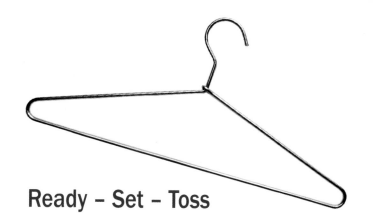

Now that you understand all the ways your clothes can connect with your own physical characteristics, we're ready to start building a wardrobe. If you've ever uttered those familiar words: "I have nothing to wear"… take heart. You are about to discover how to spend the same money, own half the clothes, and have twice as much to wear. It's much easier than you probably imagine.

Start by organizing the clothes you already own. Now that you know what colors, styles and details are most flattering, you can easily determine what items should stay and what needs to go.

Of course it isn't easy to let go of perfectly usable clothing. But when you get rid of a garment or accessory that doesn't look or feel good, you're making room in your life for one that will. Chances are you don't actually wear those misfits anyway. Some of them may have clearance tags still attached. And you can sell those discarded items online or donate them to bless some other woman in need.

You'll need to gather some supplies and look your best before you start.

- You'll want quality hangers for the items you're keeping. Take the wire ones back to the dry cleaner for recycling. They're not supporting your clothes, and they get all tangled and make you crazy anyway. See page 172 for some good options. Buy plenty—you can always return the extras.

- You'll also want cardboard boxes or trash bags labeled for categories like: Donate, Take to Recycling, Give to Sis, Take to Tailor for Alterations, Store Elsewhere.

- A garment rack is a big help, but not essential.

- You'll want sticky notes or tags to label items that need repair or alteration.

- And plan for some snacks and beverages to keep you at peak energy.

- Style your hair and put on makeup, good underwear, and pantyhose if you wear them. You're going to be trying things on, and nothing will look good if YOU look a mess.

Ready – Set – Toss

☐ **1. Remove every non-wardrobe item from your closet.** You don't need to be dodging tennis rackets, photos you're going to put in an album someday, the vacuum cleaner or anything else you don't wear, so find new homes for those other things.

☐ **2. Pull every wearable item out** of your closet, drawers, the attic, under the bed, the laundry room, and anywhere else you stash clothes—especially the ones you don't really wear. Each item needs to earn its way back into that closet.

☐ **3. Store away items that won't work for the coming season.** Trying to consider an entire year's wardrobe is just too overwhelming for most women. Focus on fall/winter or spring/summer and save the opposite season clothes for another time.

☐ **4. Group like items together.** You can make a more informed choice about those black pants when you are comparing them with your six other pairs. You can ask yourself, "How many commemorative T-shirts do I really need?" and more easily let the excess quantity go.

☐ **5. Try on each remaining item.** You can't evaluate the fit or flattery while it's on the hanger. And you may discover some forgotten treasures.

☐ **6. Try on, evaluating things using this point system:**

Design lines flatter my body shape . . . .*2 points*
Fits well . . . .*2 points*
Can be readily altered . . . .*1 point*
Flattering color . . . .*2 points*
Design details match my facial structure . . .*2 points*
In good condition . . . .*2 points*
Styling is current . . . .*2 points*
Can be easily updated . . . .*1 point*

9-12 points — a likely keeper, probably part of your new wardrobe plan. If it needs minor repairs, label it and put it in the "tailor" box. Otherwise hang it and return it to the closet.

0-4 points — an equally obvious discard. You probably don't wear it anyway. It just takes up valuable closet space and makes you feel guilty about a shopping mistake. Who needs all that negative energy? Get rid of it before you change your mind.

♦ Swap with friends. Your trash could be their treasures and vice versa.

♦ Resale shops will generally pay you half the retail they get for your items, but their standards are high. Items must be fairly new, in perfect condition, cleaned and pressed.

♦ Donate gently worn or out-of-style items to a charity or thrift shop. Be sure to get a receipt; those contributions are tax-deductible.

♦ We used to recommend throwing away the worn-out pieces. But with a reminder from the younger generation that there really is no "away" for them to go to, we now suggest checking online for a recycler in your area who accepts and reuses textiles.

5-8 points — the challenging "maybe" category. Maybe this item is a candidate for an update. Could you move it up into the keeper category by:

♦ Lengthening, shortening or tapering it for more flattering fit? (See page 194.)

♦ Dyeing it a better color? (See page 191.)

♦ Adding a trim, or removing one?

♦ Replacing unattractive buttons? (See page 192.)

♦ Combining it with a more flattering garment or accessory?

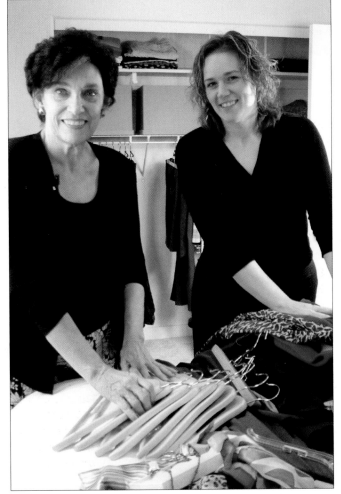

If you can't update, decide if you can discard it now, or if you need to keep it until you can afford its replacement.

Sometimes women keep clothes for pretty irrational reasons, like:

♦ **"It might come back in style."** Fashion does run in cycles, but a look seldom comes back quite the same. Our tastes—and bodies—nearly always change in the interim. Top quality fabrics and classic styles are likely to come back. Trendy prints, exaggerated trim or details, loud plaids, oversized collars, extremely wide or narrow lapels, and other unusual fashion details are rarely seen again.

♦ **"I'm going to lose weight."** Yeah, me too. But in the meanwhile neither of us needs a daily confrontation with garments that remind us we haven't done it yet. Keep them if you must, but put them in another closet, the attic or basement. And while you're at it, group and label them by the weight you need to be to wear them again.

♦ **"It has sentimental value."** Wonderful; keep it in a special sentimental spot outside your working closet. Or take a photo, snip a bit of the fabric and make a sentimental scrapbook.

If you just can't part with some of your "maybe" items, put them in a storage box or extra suitcase in the basement for now. Check them again in six months and you'll either find an unexpected treasure or a good laugh.

Style Updates

Don't hesitate to remodel even an expensive garment. Better to refit or restyle it than have it hang unworn in the spare closet gathering dust. Consider these factors:

♦ How much will the update cost? Or if you can sew, how much time will it take? If you would pay that much money or invest that much time to obtain the item new, then it is probably worth the investment to put it back into use.

♦ Is the quality of the fabric worth the update investment?

♦ Would replacing the item be easier or cheaper?

♦ Are seam allowances deep enough to let out? Will pockets or other design details get in the way of the alteration and complicate the process?

♦ Will original stitching lines or hemlines show?

We're talking here about updating clothes you already own, but the same techniques can apply to new purchases too. Frequently a nearly right item just needs minor changes to fit or look like a million. A tapered side seam, a better hemline, or classier buttons can make fashion magic.

Chapter 18 will give you the sewing techniques you need to accomplish simple updates, and give you additional ideas for makeovers with professional help.

If you need a pro to execute your restyling plans:

♦ Shop around to find someone you trust. Ask friends for recommendations, then try various seamstresses for single items and compare the results before you drop off a big group of projects.

♦ Many of the finest sewing professionals are members of the Association of Sewing and Design Professionals. You can check their website sewingprofessionals.org for a member in your area.

♦ Don't be embarrassed to ask about fees ahead of time. But don't expect quotes over the phone, especially for complicated restyling projects.

Making Basic Black Work For You

Although black isn't nearly as universally flattering as the fashion world would have you believe, most women's closets are full of it. You may be unable to—or not choose to—discard all your black right away, even if it doesn't especially flatter you. (See more about black on page 27.)

Here's a way to make that standard black suit instantly more flattering. Instead of the typical white shirt (too contrasting for nearly all women), wear it with a neutral top similar to your hair color and add an accessory that includes both colors.

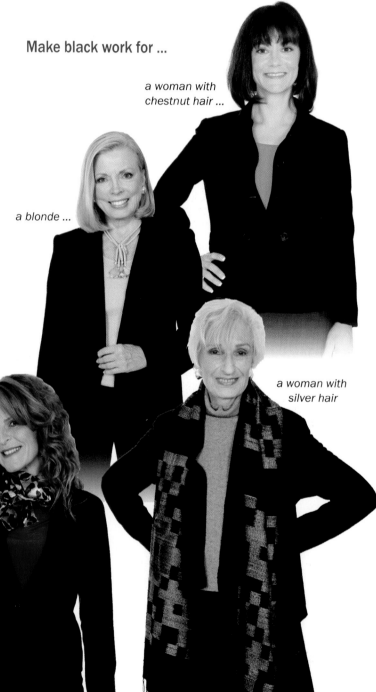

Make black work for ...

a woman with chestnut hair ...

a blonde ...

a woman with silver hair

a redhead ...

Restock Your Closet

Now hang all the keepers back in your closet. Hang everything. You're far less likely to wear items you have folded in drawers or stacked on shelves.

♦ Hang one item per hanger. That allows you to group garments by category, making any gaps in your wardrobe more obvious.

♦ Exceptions: two-piece dresses or suits you would never wear except as a unit.

♦ For slippery or stretchy garments, add peel-and-stick foam strips to the hanger to grip the shoulder area to keep them securely in place, or purchase non-slip hangers such as Huggable Hangers.

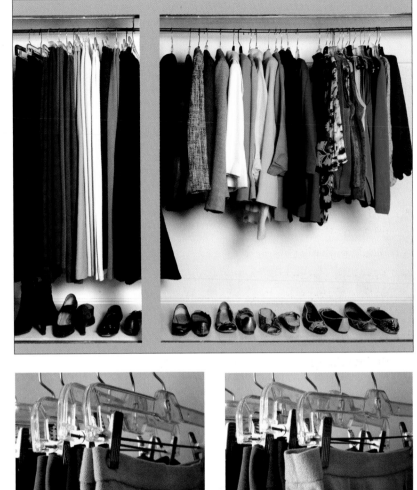

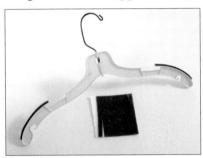

♦ For heavier sweaters, fold the garment in half along the center front/center back so one sleeve lies on top of the other. Place a hanger across the upper body area, with the hook extending from the underarm area. Fold the body down over the top edge of the hanger, then fold the sleeves down in the same way.

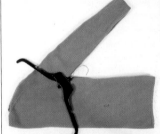

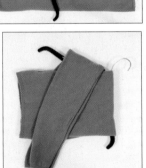

For many more tips on closet organization, see pages 170-177.

A good way to hang pants.

A less tidy way to hang pants.

♦ Use clip hangers for pants, tucking the waistline in at center front and center back so the resulting folds follow the creases in the pant leg and the garment shape is more fully supported.

♦ With everything hanging, **organize your garments by category** (jackets together, pants together, skirts together, etc.). Plan categories that fit your lifestyle. For example, you might group all pants together, or segregate career trousers from casual jeans and corduroys—it's your call.

♦ Within each category, **arrange garments in color order**: neutrals first, dark to light. Group colored pieces in rainbow order—red, orange, yellow, green, blue, purple. Arrange each color category light to dark as well. Print garments go in the grouping for their dominant color. And by the way, you'll also want every garment buttoned and facing the same direction. It may sound unnecessary now, but we're betting that a week from now you'll be a believer.

Chapter 10
Wardrobe Building

Start With Your Closet

With your closet contents edited and organized, this is the ideal time to see how many outfits you can create from the remaining pieces.

Put on the first garment from your closet—in Emmy's case it's a gray pant. Pull out the first top—a lightweight gray turtleneck, in our example—hold it up to your body and check the mirror. Could these two be worn together?

If the answer is no, return the turtleneck to the closet and move on to the next top. But if the answer is yes, put on the top and work with accessories to complete the look. What shoes? What hosiery? Does it need a belt? What about a scarf? Or jewelry? If you need inspiration, detailed information about accessories begins on page 110.

A stylish outfit typically includes three components: the bottom garment, the top garment, and the all-important "third element" that adds punch and polish to the look:

♦ An interesting pattern or texture in the top garment (or occasionally the bottom garment).

♦ An upper-body accessory—scarf, necklace, pin, silk flower, or other focal point.

♦ A jacket—more about that shortly.

If your combination needs a finishing touch you don't have, add it to your Needs List (page 96) for an upcoming shopping trip. When you are satisfied with the look, snap a picture of yourself in the mirror with a smartphone or tablet so you'll remember it. (The tablet's larger images may make shopping for coordinates easier.)

'Speed Dating' for Your Clothes

Emmy has a gray pant and sweater that she can start with. How many outfits can she create using these two pieces by changing accessories?

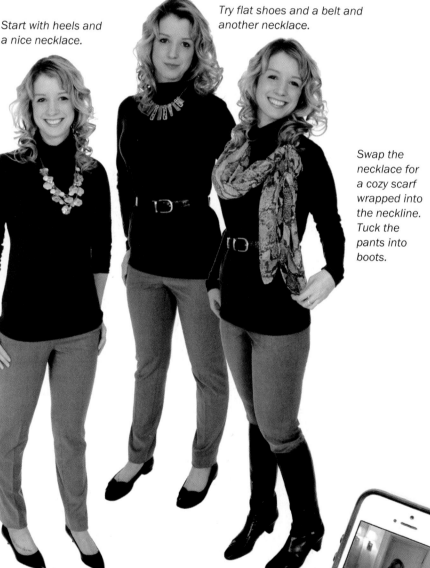

Start with heels and a nice necklace.

Try flat shoes and a belt and another necklace.

Swap the necklace for a cozy scarf wrapped into the neckline. Tuck the pants into boots.

Stand in front of a mirror and snap a picture of every combination you create.

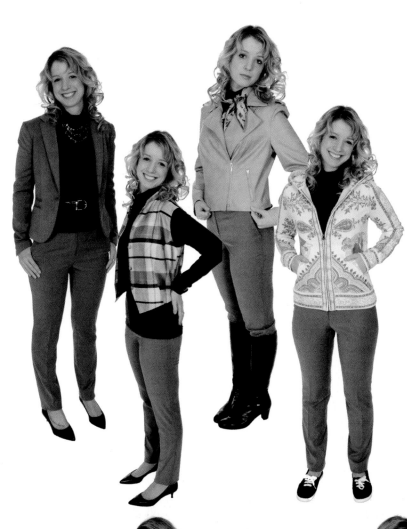

Try on Over-Layer Tops

Now before you take off the turtleneck, check the first jacket in your closet. Can it layer over this combination? NO? Then back into the closet it goes. YES? Put it on and accessorize the look, then snap a photo.

Even if you have a relaxed lifestyle and don't often wear tailored jackets, over-layer tops have some significant wardrobe advantages. They can:

- ◆ Camouflage mid-body figure challenges.
- ◆ Modify the mood of the original two-garment combination.
- ◆ Add many more mix/match options to your repertoire.

Consider these over-layer top options:

- ◆ The jacket that matches the pant
- ◆ A cardigan sweater
- ◆ A vest
- ◆ A jean jacket
- ◆ A casual shirt worn unbuttoned as a faux jacket

Try all of your remaining over-layers with the gray pants and top. Some will work, some won't.

Find a Second Top

When you've considered them all, move on to top #2. Emmy's next top is a blush pink shell. It's no accident that it blends beautifully with her gray pants. Almost any two colors from your color fan can look lovely with each other. If the combination is particularly non-traditional, add an accessory that includes both colors to "link" the look together.

When you've tried all the combinations with the gray pant, move on to the next bottom garment and repeat the process. Keep going until you've tried all the tops with all the bottoms.

You may need a break for a power bar and a beverage! This exercise may take longer than you expect—and that's GOOD NEWS. Who imagined you could find so many options from a limited number of pieces?

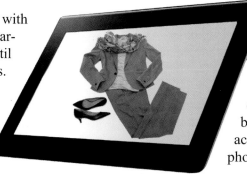

If you get tired of trying on every combination, you can use the "scarecrow" technique. Simply lay out the pieces on a plain background, add the accessories and snap your photo of that instead.

Now take a look at your dresses.

Some can be worn only one way—and that's just fine. But can some be dressed up or down by varying the accessories or adding layers?

For Emmy, the LBD is a "little BASIC dress"— not a little black one. This shade of gray balances with her soft color values and emphasizes her blue-gray eyes. It has plenty of style interest to wear on its own, accessorized for casual or dressier occasions.

The same dress works as a jumper over a long-sleeved turtleneck or tee. Black tights and black shoes elongate the silhouette.

Add the oatmeal sweater for a cozy outfit in a sophisticated mix of neutral tones. The gold/silver combo in the necklace relates to Emmy's hair and eye colors as well as the garment colors.

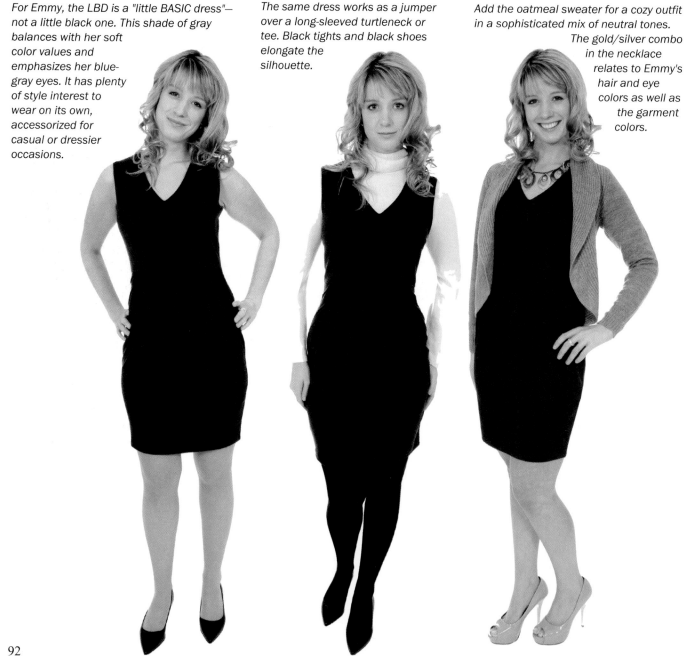

92

The dress is really a color column in one piece! With the blazer buttoned over, it creates the look of a skirt and shell.

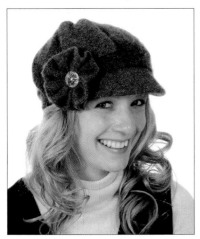

For a chilly day, Emmy finished the outfit with a patterned infinity scarf and this cute hat—a craft show find repurposed from an old cashmere sweater.

If her day at work goes into the evening, she can pull her cowl neck sweater over the top of the dress and switch out the boots for the pumps. The shirring on the sweater helps hide the dress details.

What dresses in your closet can YOU wear in multiple ways?

When You're Finished, Let's Debrief

♦ What patterns did you spot?

♦ Could you create dressier and more casual looks from the same garments by changing accessories?

♦ Were certain items more versatile than others? What styles? What fabrics? What colors?

♦ Did you find "orphans"—perfectly good pieces that you just had nothing to wear with?

♦ Did you start to fill up a Needs List of linking accessories? (See page 96.)

♦ If you found a dozen ways to use your navy trouser from your closet, did you realize you could duplicate nearly all the same combinations around a great pair of dark wash jeans? And again around a navy pencil skirt? If you don't own those items you can add them to a needs list.

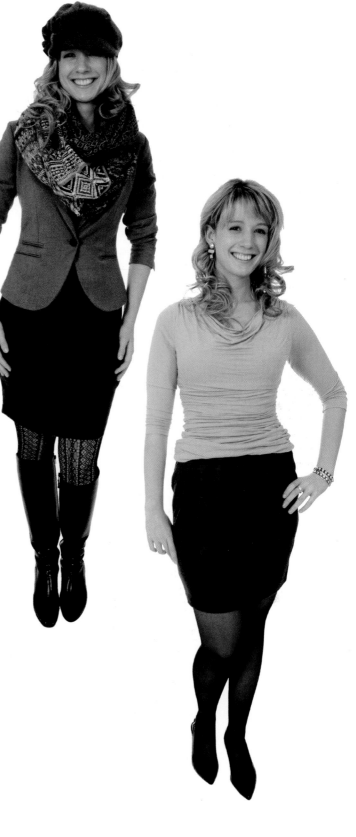

Chapter 11
The Capsule Concept

Now that you've seen how readily pieces with points of connection can work together, let's explore ways to develop the capsule formula of wardrobe development. No, that's not a pill you take to forget your fashion frustrations! It simply means building on what you already own to create groups of 5-12 related pieces that can be worn in a multitude of combinations. Our example of a 12-piece capsule starts on page 98.

There is no one formula for putting a capsule together, but here are some guidelines:

♦ Solid color pieces mix more readily than patterned ones.

♦ A few print pieces can be links connecting the solids into combinations.

♦ Simple, untrimmed styles are the most versatile, and their classic lines won't look out of style next year.

♦ Year-round or season-spanning fabrics give you the most use. This is admittedly easier to accomplish in some climates than others.

♦ No two items in a capsule should be the same style. You won't get bored with a capsule that contains both trousers and corduroy jeans and both a short, slim skirt and a longer pleated style, for example.

♦ Let go of any idea that everything has to go with everything. That's just too much pressure. If most things work with most other things, you'll have as many outfits as you need.

♦ Every item should be in your most flattering colors and shapes. Versatility is worthless if all of the combinations don't flatter YOU.

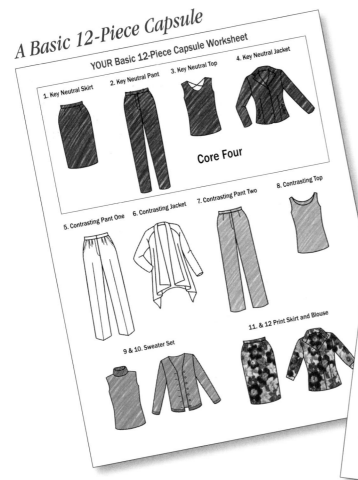

A Basic 12-Piece Capsule

YOUR Basic 12-Piece Capsule Worksheet

1. Key Neutral Skirt 2. Key Neutral Pant 3. Key Neutral Top 4. Key Neutral Jacket

Core Four

5. Contrasting Pant One 6. Contrasting Jacket 7. Contrasting Pant Two 8. Contrasting Top

9 & 10. Sweater Set 11. & 12 Print Skirt and Blouse

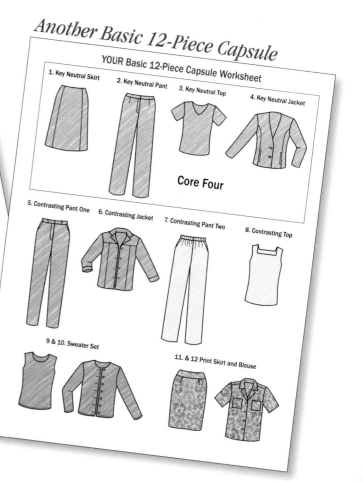

Another Basic 12-Piece Capsule

YOUR Basic 12-Piece Capsule Worksheet

1. Key Neutral Skirt 2. Key Neutral Pant 3. Key Neutral Top 4. Key Neutral Jacket

Core Four

5. Contrasting Pant One 6. Contrasting Jacket 7. Contrasting Pant Two 8. Contrasting Top

9 & 10. Sweater Set 11. & 12 Print Skirt and Blouse

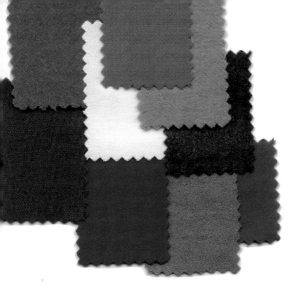

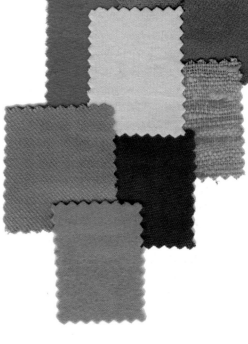

COOL	*WARM*
Black	Chocolate brown
Navy	Navy
Cherry red	Tomato red
Pearl white	Cream
Taupe	Khaki
Purple	Plum
Gray	Camel/tan
Royal blue	Teal blue

♦ Matching multiple pieces in the same solid color—even black—can be challenging. If a skirt, pant and jacket need to match, it's easiest to buy them at the same time from the same manufacturer.

♦ Recognize that those solids don't have to match exactly. Fashionable European women have long understood tonal blends and consider Americans unnecessarily "matchy-matchy." Blend one reddish brown with a slightly lighter reddish brown, but not with a golden brown, for example.

There are also a few Don'ts:

♦ Don't select stand-alone items for a capsule. A jacket with multicolor braid or contrast piping and buttons may ultimately have a place in your closet, but it probably won't play well with many other pieces in your capsule group.

♦ Don't invest your money in a style that is so "in" this year that by next year it will look undeniably "last year." (If it's truly a perfect look for you, buy it for this year, then put it away until the fad has faded from memory. Then you can bring it out and enjoy it without looking dated.)

Year-Round Colors

Seasonality of a garment is defined more by its fabric than by its color. In the year-round fabrics listed below, any of the colors above should look equally right in warm or cool weather. Of course you'll want to choose any color in the specific value and intensity from your personal color fan.

Year-Round Fabrics

You'll get the most versatile capsules using items you can wear across the seasons. Of course you'll need some pieces in your closet specifically for temperature extremes and seasonal activities. But get maximum mileage from fabrics like these:

♦ lightweight wool gabardine
♦ wool crepe
♦ rayon challis
♦ rayon-blend gabardine or crepe
♦ silk or synthetic matte jersey
♦ silk suitings
♦ silk and silk-like blouse weights
♦ cotton and cotton-blend knits
♦ cotton and cotton-blend shirtings
♦ denim and chino
♦ fine-gauge knits

Needs List

ITEM	HAVE	NEED
Key Neutral bottom garment		
Key Neutral bottom garment		
Key Neutral under-layer top		
Key Neutral over-layer top		
Secondary neutral bottom garment		
Secondary neutral under-layer top		
Dark accent color bottom garment		
Matching dark accent color over-layer top		
Accent color twin tops		
Accent color over-layer top		
Accent color under-layer top		
Accent color under-layer top		
Accent color under-layer top		
Accent color under-layer top		
Patterned bottom		
Patterned top		
Key Neutral casual shoe		
Key Neutral dress shoe		
Key Neutral belt		
Key Neutral handbag		
Linking accessory		
Linking accessory		
Linking accessory		
Linking accessory		

Needs List

Regardless of lifestyle, almost everyone's wardrobe is most versatile when it includes certain key components. Compare the current contents of your closet against this suggested list to identify gaps you may need to fill. Use your color fan to guide your color selections. Adapt the specific garment choices based on how formally or casually you like to dress.

♦ Your basic pant, for instance, might be corduroy jeans or it might be fine wool gabardine trousers.

♦ Your second bottom might be a skirt, another pant, capris or shorts.

♦ Your twin sweater set might be a classic shell and cardigan, or it might be a camisole and cascade-front sweater or some other pair of color-matched tops.

You may ultimately want more depth in some of these categories; this is just a starting point. And you may need specialty items for sports, cold weather, formal events, and so on. Add those to the blank lines of the chart.

Before you set out to find the items on your needs list, check pages 159-169 for smart shopping strategies.

YOUR Basic 12-Piece Capsule

On the next page is a planning worksheet you can use to create a basic 12-Piece Capsule.

Photocopy the page and use colored pencils to try out combinations for your capsule wardrobe using the shades from your color fan. You can even personalize it by copying and pasting other garment styles from the Fashion Dictionary on pages 156-158, like we have done on the worksheet samples on page 94. Typically, no two items in a capsule would be exactly the same style. But if a particular style fits and flatters you more than any other, go ahead and repeat it.

Starting on page 98 you can see how the 12 pieces in a capsule wardrobe can be combined using navy garments as your starting point.

YOUR Basic 12-Piece Capsule Worksheet

1. Key Neutral Skirt

2. Key Neutral Pant

3. Key Neutral Top

4. Key Neutral Jacket

Core Four

5. Contrasting Pant One

6. Contrasting Jacket

7. Contrasting Pant Two

8. Contrasting Top

9. & 10. Sweater Set

11. & 12. Print Skirt and Blouse

Creating New Capsules

The Basic 12-Piece Capsule

Some situations call for building a capsule from scratch rather than working from existing garments:

♦ Significant weight loss
♦ Major job change
♦ Retirement
♦ Relocating to a different climate
♦ Lifestyle change

Here is a formula for just 12 garments that can yield up to 96 outfits. Of course you'll adapt these specific garment examples to your own lifestyle and body type.

Core Four

Start with a *core four* grouping. That's a skirt, pant, blouse or shell, and jacket in the same neutral color.

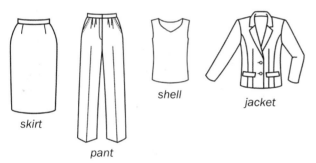

skirt

pant

shell

jacket

These four navy pieces make four complete outfits:

♦ Skirt and shell
♦ Pant and shell
♦ Skirt, shell, jacket
♦ Pant, shell, jacket

This monochromatic look requires emphatic accessories to keep it fresh and interesting. But—more important—these four pieces create four different color columns. A color column is an unbroken vertical flow of color from top to bottom of a look. Your core four create these columns:

♦ Skirt and shell—an inside column
♦ Pant and shell—an inside column
♦ Pant and jacket—an outside column
♦ Skirt and jacket—an outside column

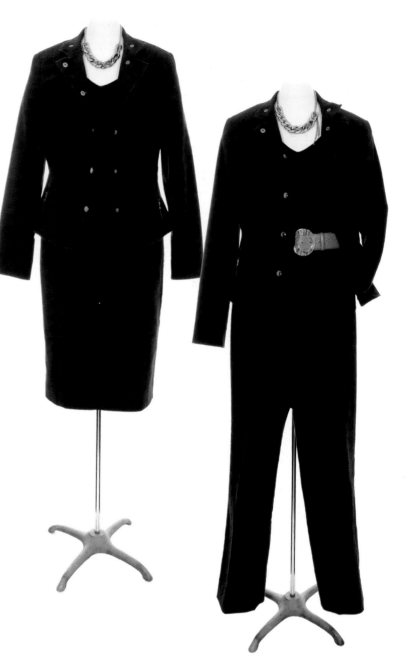

inside color columns

outside color columns

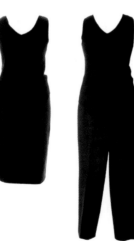
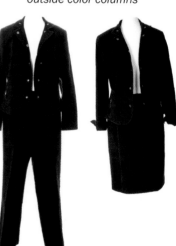

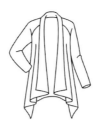 **You can layer a contrasting blouse or shell under either of the outside columns—** and a link to connect the colors. Of course the shell can also work with the bottoms— no jacket required.

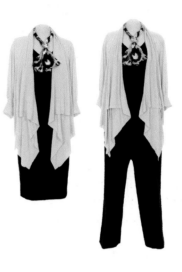 **You can also layer a contrast jacket over the inside columns** and connect with a link. We used a cream sweater.

Add a bottom to match the cream sweater for a new outside column. Layer in the taupe or navy top. You could also wear the pants-and-top combinations without the sweater.

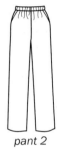

NOTE: What looks like a new navy top is actually our original tank worn backwards to show off the back design detail— try it with knit tops in your own wardrobe!

pant 2

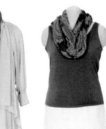

Add a bottom to match the contrast shell for another inside column.

Top that with either jacket.

pant 3

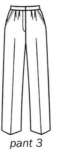

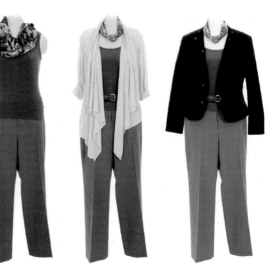

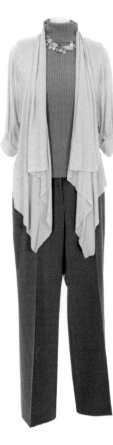

A twin sweater set is a useful addition to the grouping. It might be a traditional shell and cardigan or a more creative style. Either way, the set works with all four bottoms in the grouping. Since this mix breaks up your *color columns*, be sure the link repeats the bottom garment color near the top of the look for visual continuity.

twin sweater set

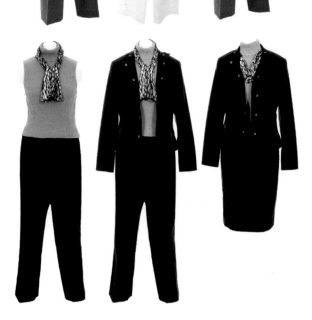

The shell from the sweater set works with any of the bottoms, either as a stand-alone or under either jacket.

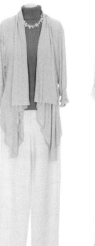

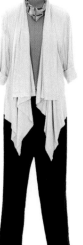

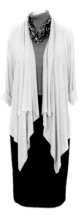

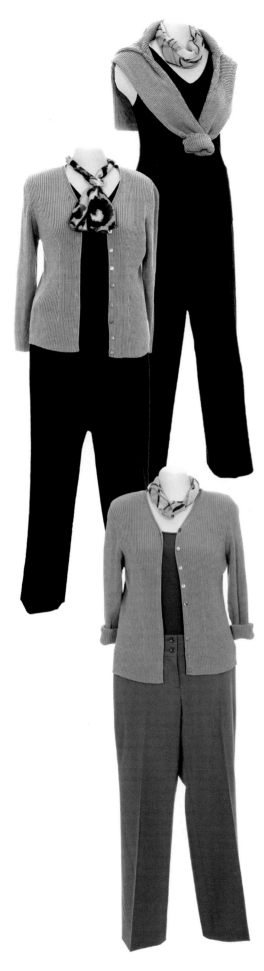

The cardigan can be worn (or tied) over each of the color columns, and worn over any mix of the other tops and bottoms.

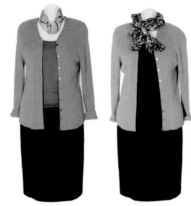

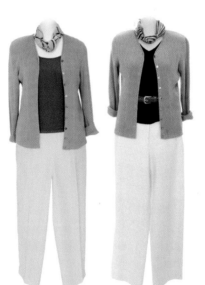

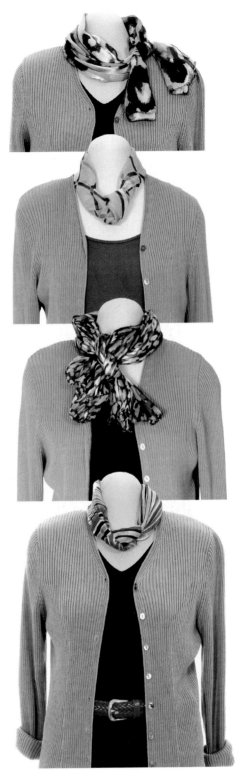

Linking accessories are especially important to keep three-color combinations cohesive. See pages 119-125 for easy ways to tie a scarf. Or look for a necklace or earrings that include all the capsule colors.

Next add a print blouse in the colors of the separates.

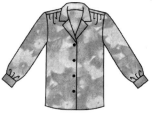

- Layer it under any of the three outside columns.
- Wear it as a single layer with any of the bottoms. We've shown it here with the navy pant.
- Or wear it unbuttoned as a lightweight jacket over the inside columns like the taupe combination below.
- The print becomes a link for combining any of the solid pieces. The navy pant and taupe shell shown below is just one example. How many more can you find?

Sneaky tip: If you start your capsule by finding a great print made up of colors from your color fan, it will automatically define the solids for the other pieces of the grouping.

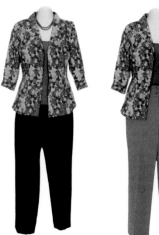

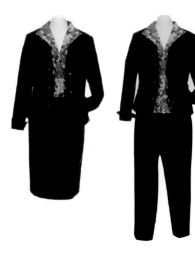

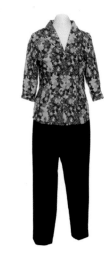

Finally, add a skirt in the matching print.

Worn with the blouse, it gives the look of a dress.

- Wear the dress solo or top it with the jacket or either cardigan.
- Wear the skirt with the twin set.
- Or with the periwinkle shell and any over-layer top. We chose the cream sweater.
- Or with the navy shell and any over-layer top, including the print shirt.
- Or with the taupe shell and any of the over-layer tops.

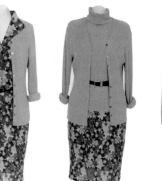

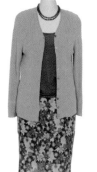

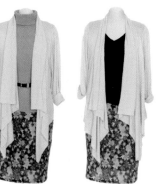

If every piece works with every other piece, this 12-piece grouping can yield an astonishing 96 combinations. You may not care for every possible combination. That's fine. If your 12-piece grouping yields only 82 outfits or 68 or just 52—whatever—it will almost certainly be more versatile than the wardrobe you had before. You can choose your combination for any given day based on the dressiness of your activities, the weather, your mood and—let's be honest here—what's not in the laundry.

Accessorizing Your Capsule

Wardrobe capsules help you get maximum mileage from accessories too.

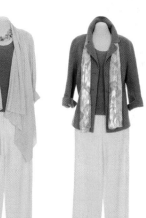

The sample capsule on the previous pages requires only:

♦ Navy flats and pumps
♦ Taupe low-heeled pumps
♦ Taupe and red belts
♦ Taupe and navy bags
♦ Six scarves in capsule colors
♦ Four fashion jewelry sets

See Chapter 12 for much more information about choosing accessories.

Add a Few More Pieces

Of course you probably don't want to spend every day in the same three or four colors. And you'll almost certainly want more than 12 garments in your closet. Another set of matching tops is a great way to add variety. We chose a hot pink unlined jacket and matching knit shell and immediately found 10 new outfits, including these:

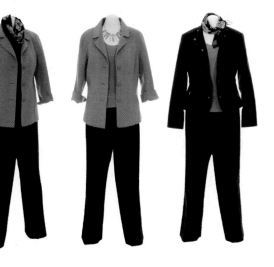

Want Even More Variety?

◆ Jade green would be another great accent color to add. A simple shell would give an entirely different look to the outside columns of navy or cream.

◆ Print or plaid pieces in any mix of your colors would make great additions, too.

◆ A *core four* (jacket, pant, skirt, and top—page 98) in medium gray would coordinate with nearly all the existing pieces in cream, periwinkle, taupe, and even navy.

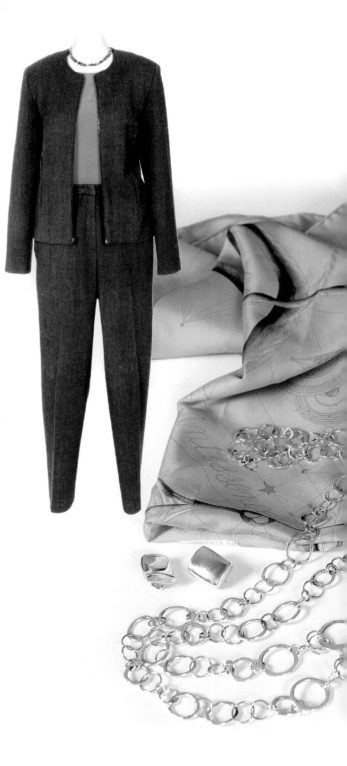

◆ The solid colors and streamlined styles at the heart of the capsule concept make the ideal backdrop for WOW pieces—vintage, eclectic, wearable art, designer—that showcase your personal style and add pizzazz to your wardrobe.

This vintage Hmong appliquéd and embroidered batik jacket picks up the capsule colors and makes a very personal statement, even when combined with traditional colors and garment styles.

◆ A great pair of dark wash jeans can work with all the top combinations to create a range of more casual looks.

A Casual Capsule

Many women put all their attention into career wardrobes and have virtually nothing nice to wear in their private lives. Fortunately, the capsule concept works just as well with very casual styles and fabrics.

A casual capsule—even using a less precise plan and choosing more patterned pieces—can give you stylish choices for family and social time without breaking the bank.

Of course your own casual capsule will reflect your personal coloring and your style preference. Ours was built around some summer sportswear standards—white jeans, denim shorts, railroad stripe capris, a cotton cardigan, striped tee and a pair of soft knit camisoles. Then for fun we added a border print skirt, mini-print tiered cami and a dressed-up sweatshirt jacket for chilly evenings.

We found nearly 30 combinations—some of which are pictured here. Notice how the necklace links the teal cami, white pants and red cardigan into a striking, unexpected combination.

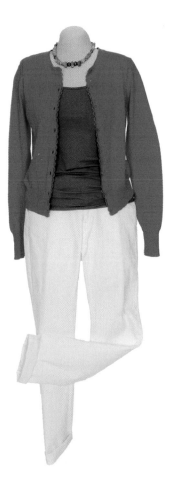

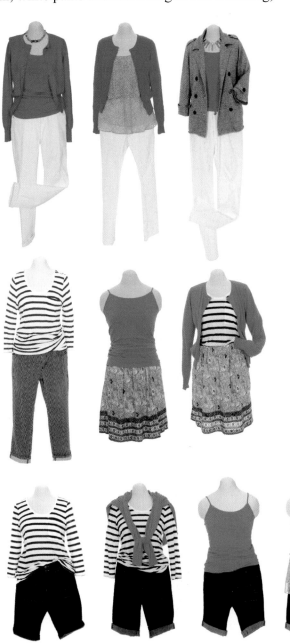

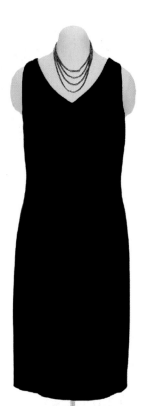

An Evening Capsule

Dressy social occasions are a major wardrobe challenge for many women. We love to look special, but find it frustrating to spend big bucks for a knock-out, wear-it-once garment. (See cost-per-wearing formula, page 161.)

Capsule groupings are the answer once again. A carefully selected group of separates can take you through a decade of dressy affairs without anyone thinking "She wore that last year."

Choose late-day fabrics like crepe de chine, crepe-back satin, silk jersey, velvet, satin, brocade, and metallics. Add a new item or two each year and you'll never regard a dressy event as a closet crisis again.

Dress for not-quite-so-formal occasions by mixing your evening capsule items with pieces from your regular wardrobe. For example, the silk camisole and glitzy earrings can dress up a collarless wool crepe suit for a holiday business event. The brocade jacket can top gabardine trousers and a silky blouse for a festive open house.

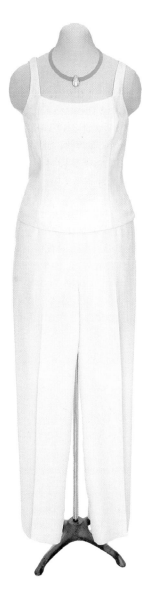

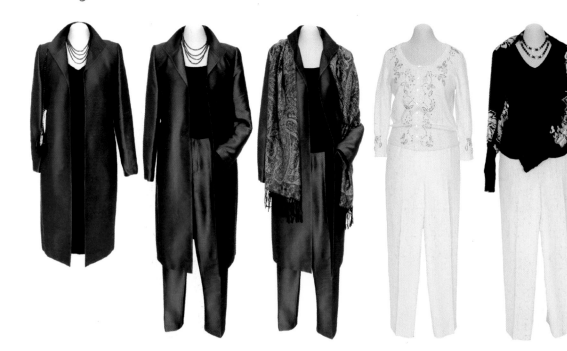

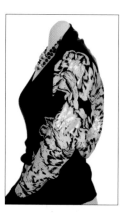

See page 123 for more about using a scarf as a shrug.

Don't overlook the accessories for your dressy capsule. You can ruin a dressy look with a clunky leather shoe or your everyday handbag. Or, in reverse, you can take the crepe suit look up another notch with a jeweled peau de soie shoe and a metallic evening clutch.

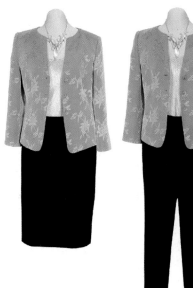

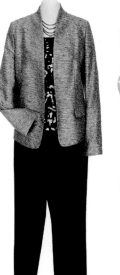

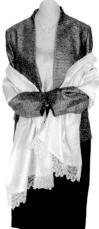

Mixing Textures

Designers use unexpected texture contrasts to add elegant individuality. Mixing textures is easier than mixing patterns. Here are some guidelines:

♦ Medium textures are easiest to work with. They combine well with one another and with smooth or highly textured surfaces as well. Soft flannel trousers, for example, can blend with a satin blouse or with a sweater-knit jacket.

♦ Extreme textures combine easily if they are in the same mood. For example, wool tweed mixes easily with suede; satin blends readily with sequins.

♦ Mixing extreme textures of different mood typically creates an eclectic, offbeat feeling.

Mixing It Up With Prints and Textures

Mix prints, or prints with plaids? Why of course! Men do it every day when they combine subtly patterned suits, shirts and ties. Designers like Koos Van Den Akker and Missoni have built international reputations on it. And patchwork quilts raise print mixing to an art form.

Although you can create any combination that pleases you, here are some guidelines to consider:

♦ Pattern mixes are most understandable when the patterns relate to one another either in the design shapes or in the colorations.

♦ If the colors are different, the repeated design shapes provide the visual connection. A preppy patchwork of madras plaids is an obvious example of this concept.

♦ If the print motifs are not similar, repeated colors tie the look together. A mix of dots and stripes in the same colors is a simple example of this look. A print blouse in the same colors as a tweed jacket takes this concept to a more complex level.

♦ Unexpected mixes become more understandable when the two patterns vary in scale. If one print has large shapes, try accenting it with another, smaller pattern. A small pattern can often function as a semisolid, just one with more visual interest.

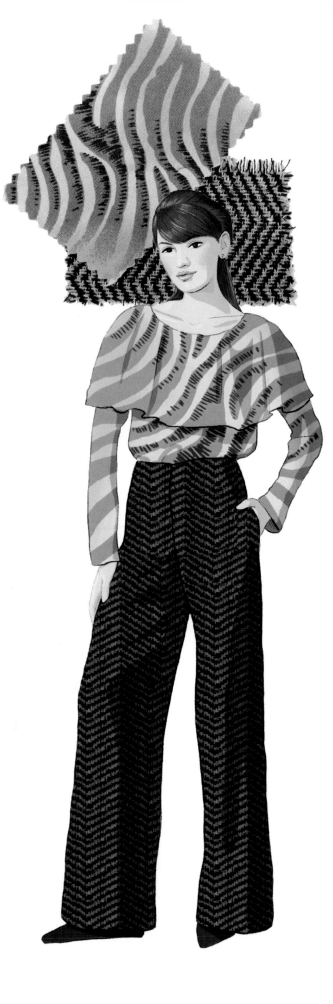

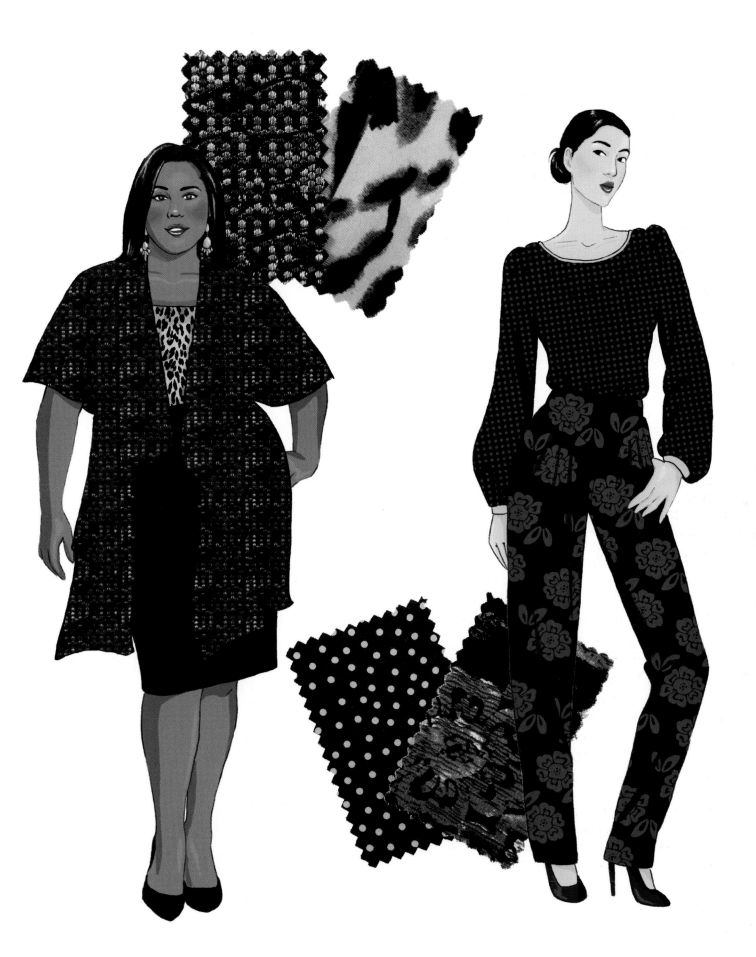

Chapter 12

Accessory Connections

The Accessory Advantage

Accessories can be the glue that holds your wardrobe together, linking separate garments into fashion-right ensembles. They are great wardrobe extenders because they create the illusion that you are wearing a different outfit every day. And they have the ability to carry a combination of garments up or down the formality scale over a range of events and activities.

Wardrobe consultants often guide clients to spend as much as a third of their wardrobe budget on accessories. They are a wise investment because most accessories last years longer than most garments. And they usually aren't affected by your weight and size variations either. Did you ever hear anyone say, "I've gained weight and can't squeeze into my scarf"?

So invest in the best accessories you can afford, choosing items that maximize points of connection with your color fan, body scale, facial structure and facial scale. Good pieces are always in style. It's better to avoid spending on faddish pieces that are ultimately just "throwaway chic."

Use those accessories to:

♦ link unexpected combinations of your best colors into sophisticated outfits.

♦ give new punch to a wardrobe classic.

♦ transform an outfit instantly from a daytime look to after-five.

♦ focus attention at the parts of your body you'd like to have noticed, and away from any perceived challenges.

♦ add color and energy to combinations of neutral garments.

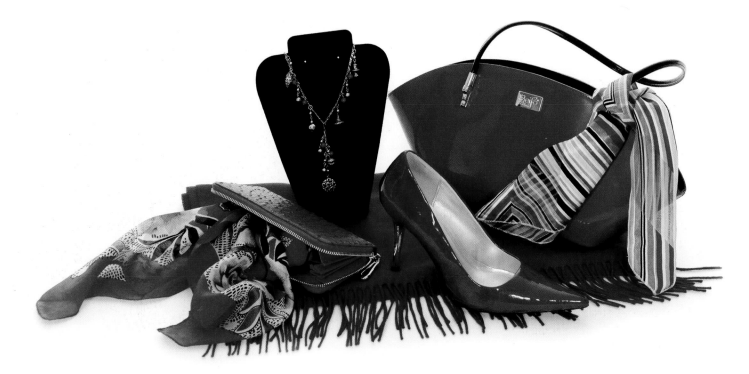

Shoes and Hose

First and foremost, footwear must be comfortable. It's tough to present an appealing look if your face is contorted in pain. But within the range of what you find comfortable, you can certainly find options that are also attractive.

Leather is the best investment for comfort and durability. It molds its shape to your foot, and its porous nature allows perspiration to evaporate, keeping your feet cool and dry. Patent leather's shiny finish is more popular for warm-weather wear, while suede's soft brushed texture is typically limited to cool-weather seasons.

Manmade look-alikes come in a variety of quality levels and more affordable price points. Shoes with fabric uppers provide a wide range of color choices, but typically have a shorter life and need a waterproofing treatment to resist stains.

Considering the cost of better leather goods, your selections should work with almost everything in your wardrobe. Shop with your color fan and keep your personal style and facial structure (page 76) -in mind.

Best Bets to Buy

♦ The most basic shoe for most women is a low-heeled closed-toe pump in your key neutral—typically a color closely related to your hair color. This classic style works with both pants and skirts. Basic pumps need not be boring—interesting trim details or mixed materials can add lots of visual interest.

♦ Although many stylists consider black to be the universal neutral, it isn't a great shoe choice if it isn't part of your personal color fan. Your hair color, on the other hand, is always part of your total look. Presumably any wardrobe color you'd choose would harmonize with your hair, and therefore with hair-color shoes too.

♦ If your hair color is very pale blonde or silver gray you may prefer a darker version of that color for basic footwear. Rich tans or medium grays would be good options.

♦ Another option is to match the shoe to the color of your skirt or pant—a practical approach when the garment is a neutral. This applies especially to navy. Women with warm coloring, who wear warmer shades of navy, will prefer navy leather shoes. Because the navy color is applied to warm tan natural leather, the result is a warm shade of navy. Women who wear a cool navy will find a better match with shoes made from microfiber fabric or leather-look synthetic material.

♦ Shoe color should usually be a similar value or darker than your bottom garment to ground the look and avoid calling too much attention to the feet.

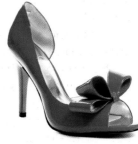

♦ Bright contrasting colors and highly embellished or multicolor shoes form a focal point low on the body and create a shorter, stockier appearance. If you choose bright, contrast shoes, try repeating the color near the top of the ensemble—as a necklace, scarf or pin, for example—to balance the look. The accessory capsule on the previous pages is an example.

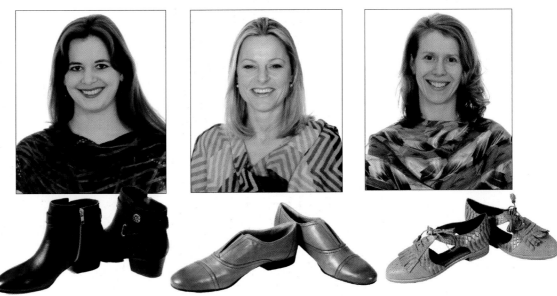

- With a skirt, a lower vamp (top opening of the shoe) leaves more of your foot visible and elongates your legs.

- Peep-toe and sling-back styles that expose more skin have a similar visual impact.

- The more skin a shoe exposes, the less appropriate it is for a traditional business setting.

- With pants, a higher vamp brings the shoe color up to meet the pants hem, avoiding a distracting band of exposed skin.

- Avoid ankle strap styles unless you have very long, trim legs and can afford their shortening, widening effect.

- Lighter-weight styling and higher, thinner heels make a shoe dressier.

- Heavier material, thicker soles and shorter, thicker heels move the styling in a more casual direction.

- Wedge styling provides more support than other heel designs of similar height. This style has a more casual feeling when the wedge is covered with cork or jute, a more professional feeling with a matching leather wedge.

- Evening shoes are typically made from dressy fabrics like satin and peau de soie. Only the most delicate leather high-heeled sandals can look correct with after-five clothing.

- Even comfort shoes can be stylish. Brands like Clarks, Dansko, Naot, Naturalizer, and Ros Hommerson, among others, offer special comfort features in an array of styles and colors.

- Athletic shoes belong in true sports environments. For very relaxed outfits, a lightweight canvas sneaker is a more stylish and flattering choice.

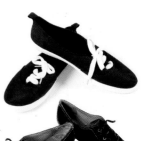

- A new athletic shoe designed to go with casual clothes is called a "lifestyle shoe."

Boots

In colder climates, classic boots in quality leather are a good investment. Your key neutral is usually the most versatile color choice. Many women have had trouble finding boots wide enough to accommodate their calf, but newer styles are now available to meet that need. Some online footwear retailers even include a search criteria for calf circumference measurement. Shoe repair professionals can also expand the top of a narrow boot to fit your leg.

When wearing boots with a skirt, you can create the longest, leanest look when the skirt hem covers the boot top. Matching tights can help avoid having skin visible as you walk. Tights also make it easier to look slim wearing shorter or ankle-length boots with skirts. Just as with a regular shoe, the height and thickness of the heel indicates the dressiness of a boot. Lower, chunkier heels denote practicality; higher, thinner heels are typically a dressier look.

Choose additional shoes based on your lifestyle and your personal style. The chart below presents some options.

	Evening	Casual	Sports
Tailored Classic	peau de soie pump with gold trim	tassled walker	sneakers
Feminine Romantic	strappy sandal	bowed ballet flat	sneakers
High-Fashion Dramatic	jeweled 3" heel	patchwork metallic slip-on	sneakers
Artistic	ruby slippers	vintage western boots	hand-painted sneakers
Sporty	plain peau de soie	penny loafers	sneakers

Hosiery and Tights

Once considered an essential component of women's professional and dressy attire, sheer nude hosiery is now at the center of a fashion debate. Some stylists dismiss it as inherently dowdy and un-sophisticated, while most career counselors consider it part of the essential physical boundaries women must set in the workplace. Here's our take on the subject:

♦ In conservative professions like law and finance, hosiery is generally expected when wearing a skirt in most climates.

♦ In more relaxed work environments, bare legs and sandals can be acceptable if your dress code permits it, your legs are in great shape, and your feet freshly pedicured.

♦ With formal and cocktail attire, bare legs are acceptable for the young, toned and pedicured. Ultra-sheer hosiery with a subtle sheen is a fashionable alternative for those who prefer coverage. There are even open-toe panty hose (they have a little strip that fits between your first and second toe to keep them in place) that give a barefoot look with evening sandals while masking less than perfect legs.

New body-shaper panty hose styles contain a hefty percentage of spandex fiber. Many women love their ability to smooth and firm hips and thighs. Better than older control-top styles, they diminish the percentage of spandex gradually from waist to toe rather than ending abruptly right in the soft mid-thigh area, which created an unattractive bulge.

Colored hosiery moves in and out of fashion prominence, but matching shoes and hose to hemline color does minimize color breaks and lend a taller, trimmer look to a skirt ensemble. Here are guidelines for that look:

♦ With a garment in a neutral color like black, navy, dark brown or taupe, you can match all three color elements. Keep the hosiery very sheer for professional or dressy looks.

♦ Even sheer colored hose can seem too heavy in warmer weather, so opt for nude hosiery through the summer months.

♦ With a fashion-color suit or dress, choose either a color-matched shoe or a neutral shoe color related to your hair color. In either case, keep the hosiery neutral.

♦ With two-toned spectator shoes or multicolor print or patchwork shoes, choose nude hosiery.

♦ Off-white hose give a sort of Alice-in-Wonderland look, too girlish for adult women.

♦ Patterned, textured, lacy and fishnet stockings all draw attention to your legs and tend to make them appear heavier.

♦ Opaque tights give an outfit a casual mood; wear them with flats, boots or other chunky shoes rather than with dressy heels.

♦ With pants, fine-gauge trouser socks are another good option. Some women have fun coordinating subtly patterned socks with their outfit.

When you find a style or brand of hosiery you love, buy them in quantity, then keep a spare pair in your desk drawer and another in your car's glove compartment for emergencies.

Keep panty hose with minor runs to wear under pants if you like, but tie them in a soft knot after laundering so you can identify them easily in your lingerie drawer.

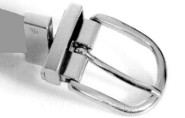

Belt Basics

♦ Leather belts in widths from ½" to 1½" are fashion classics worth collecting in all your best neutrals. Look for buckles that relate to the curve or angularity of your facial features. See page 76.

♦ Replace the fabric-covered or synthetic belts that sometimes come with dresses. Quality leather belts create a more sophisticated look.

♦ Look for great belts on sale, even if they are too long. A shoe repair shop can inexpensively remove the buckle and trim away the excess length. The shop can also recycle a favorite buckle from an old belt and attach it to a new one.

♦ Belts should be long enough to fit comfortably when buckled into the second hole.

♦ Belts that match or blend with the color of your garment are less eye-catching and give the illusion of a longer body line.

♦ Contrasting, embellished or decorative belts add more visual interest—a plus if your waistline is a figure asset you want to showcase.

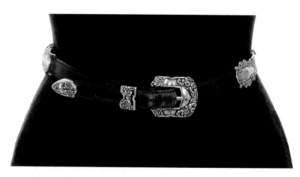

♦ Wider belts are more comfortable in softer leathers. They work best on figures with a long torso and high bust with limited waist shaping.

♦ Matching a belt to your blouse color can elongate a short-waited figure. Matching the belt color to skirt or pants can minimize a long-waisted silhouette.

♦ Contour belts—ones cut on a curve rather than straight—rest on the high hip rather than right at the waist so the torso appears longer and trimmer.

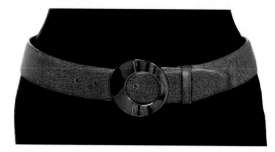

♦ A bold decorative buckle draws attention to the center of the body, creating the illusion of a narrower waist. The effect is more pronounced when the belt is worn under an open jacket.

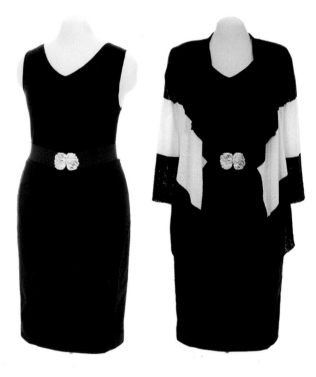

♦ A too-long belt can also be worn with the excess length wrapped back on itself in a casual look.

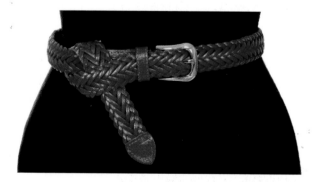

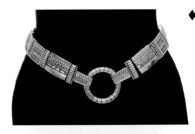

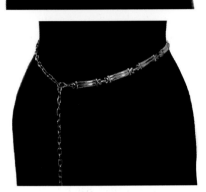

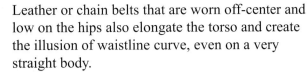

♦ Leather or chain belts that are worn off-center and low on the hips also elongate the torso and create the illusion of waistline curve, even on a very straight body.

A traditional belt, makes Cindy's waist look wide; worn at a downward angle it gives the illusion of more waistline curve and a trimmer silhouette.

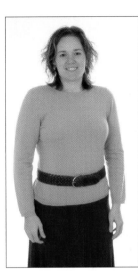

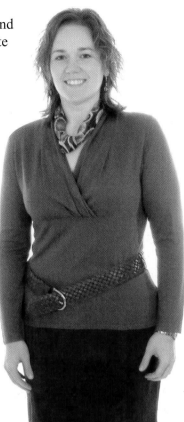

♦ This little black purse has a detachable strap that can be used as a single or double belt.

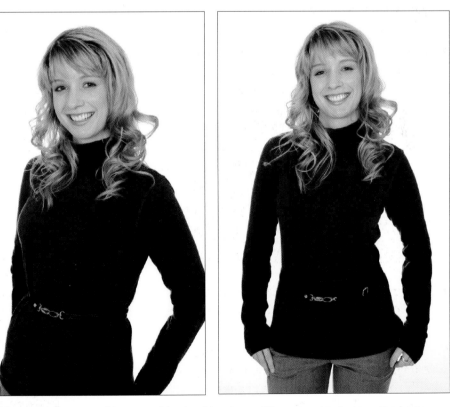

Many purses come with removable shoulder straps. When you plan to carry the bag instead, you can un-clip the strap and wear it as a coordinating belt. Adjust the length to fit your waist, to fit the belt loops of low-rise pants, or even to double-wrap over a sweater.

Handbag Basics

You wear your handbag every day, so it makes sense to choose carefully. Since you will probably use your basic bag with a very wide variety of outfits, it makes sense to keep it fairly basic—not heavily embellished and neither overly dressy or overly casual. Here are some guidelines:

♦ Although it is no longer expected that your shoes and bag will match, they should be in the same color family.

♦ Like shoes, your most basic bag color relates closely to your hair. Since your hair is always part of your total look, and presumably every wardrobe color you wear looks good with that hair color, it's logical that a bag in that color will blend with all your outfits.

♦ Additional neutrals to consider—if they appear in your color fan—include:

COOL—black, taupe, gray, navy
WARM—brown, camel, rust

Handbag Tips

♦ Look for a style with minimal, tasteful embellishment.

♦ Strong or cute prints, patchwork effects, fringe, and oversized metal hardware are so eye-catching they make the handbag a statement of its own rather than part of a beautifully integrated ensemble. Bags of this type are fine for special situations, but less practical for everyday use.

♦ Coordinate the bag's shape with the degree of curve or angularity in your facial features. See page 76.

♦ Leather—or a synthetic that looks convincingly like leather—is the most versatile choice for year-round use. In warm weather, neutral colors of canvas or straw give a fresh look and blend with virtually any shoe color.

♦ Make sure any bag you're considering has the capacity you need. Empty the contents in your current purse into the new one to test its functionality before you buy.

♦ Match a purse to your body scale with this easy test. Hold the bag in front of your pelvic area. It should generally be no wider than your hips and no taller than the distance from your waist to the crease at the top of your leg.

♦ A shoulder bag is a convenient hands-free option. Be sure the strap length positions the bag at a flattering spot on your body. If the strap isn't adjustable, a shoe repair shop can alter it to the most flattering length.

For a curved figure, the bag should rest in the waist area, not lower where it would add width to the hips

For a straighter figure, the bag should rest in the hip area to avoid adding bulk at the waist.

- Cross-body bags provide extra security—especially when traveling—but the strap worn diagonally across your torso often interferes with the drape of your clothing or outlines the bustline in an unflattering way.

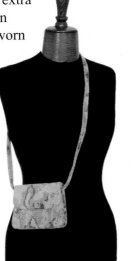

Briefcases

Professional women often need to carry papers, files and other business paraphernalia in an efficient and attractive way. Boxy, mannish briefcases are less popular today than more feminine alternatives.

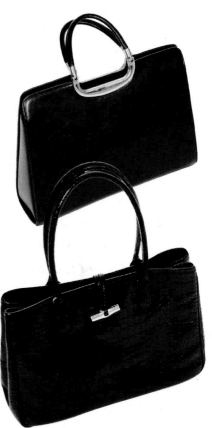

- A moderately structured portfolio is a stylish option. Choose a leather model in a darker version of your hair color to blend with your wardrobe colors.

More Handbag Types

- This handbag style is another classic. Often the straps are long enough to slip over your shoulder for added convenience and safety.

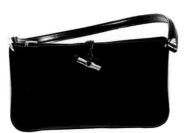

- Envelope and clutch bags provide a dressier look, ideal for a career woman to slip into a brief-case or portfolio rather than carrying two separate bags.

- For after-five events a small evening bag is simply a must. Buy a dressy fabric bag in your key neutral or a little clutch in your best metallic and use it for decades.

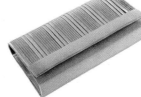

- A leather tote carried over your shoulder is a more informal look—great for more relaxed career environments.

- Consider owning a second portfolio in lighter-colored canvas or woven straw for warm weather.

Look for practical details, such as:

- detachable strap for easy carrying when hands are full.

- double stitching, reinforced handles, and metal or leather corners for durability and longer wear.

- inside compartments for organization.

- sturdy clasps or top zipper for security.

Accessory Links

Multicolor accessories—scarves and jewelry—play a powerful role in your wardrobe by linking unexpected solid colors into stunning combinations. Almost any two (or even three) colors from your personal color fan can be worn together. But the more unexpected the pairing, the more you need a link to tell people "it's an outfit—not just the only shirt I had clean this morning." Here are some examples of color combinations and the links that make them work:

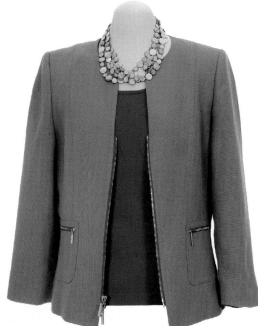

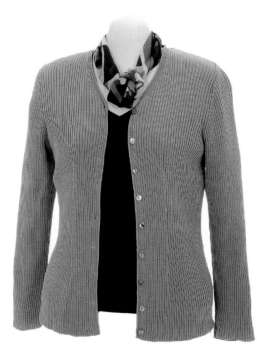

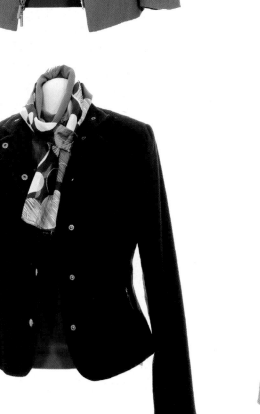

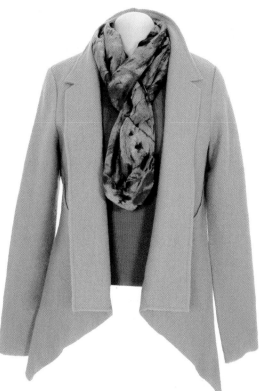

Scarf Savvy

Scarves really are wardrobe magicians. They can add instant polish and pizzazz to almost any outfit. They can link unexpected color combinations into sophisticated ensembles. They can bridge a less-flattering color to your facial color pattern. They form a powerful focal point near your face, pulling attention away from any figure challenges. And they almost never wear out, so you can enjoy your investment for years.

Be sure to carefully clip off the tag before you first wear the scarf. Save the tag if you need a reminder of the care instructions.

Keep these points in mind when you shop for scarves:

◆ Multicolor print scarves that combine several shades from your color fan are the most useful in your wardrobe. A print that includes a touch of your hair color will be especially flattering.

◆ The scale and the curve/angularity of the print motifs are less critical, since they will be obscured in the fabric folds as you tie the scarf.

◆ Silk scarves tie easily and drape softly. Silk-like polyester scarves have a crisper hand and the added advantages of wrinkle resistance and easy washability.

◆ Cotton scarves have a more casual mood, more appropriate with sportswear or jeans than with dressier clothing.

◆ Wool and rayon challis scarves look great in cool weather, but can be bulky to tie.

◆ Oblong scarves (about 15" x 60") are by far the most versatile shape, followed by small squares (14-16").

◆ Large squares (24"-36") are beautiful, but less user-friendly. Try folding them into a rectangular shape before you tie them.

◆ Pashminas—big rectangular shawls in solids or tapestry patterns—can even substitute for a jacket in spring and fall. See page 125 for tips on wearing these.

◆ An infinity scarf is a continuous loop of fabric that is easy to drape in a variety of ways. No tying required!

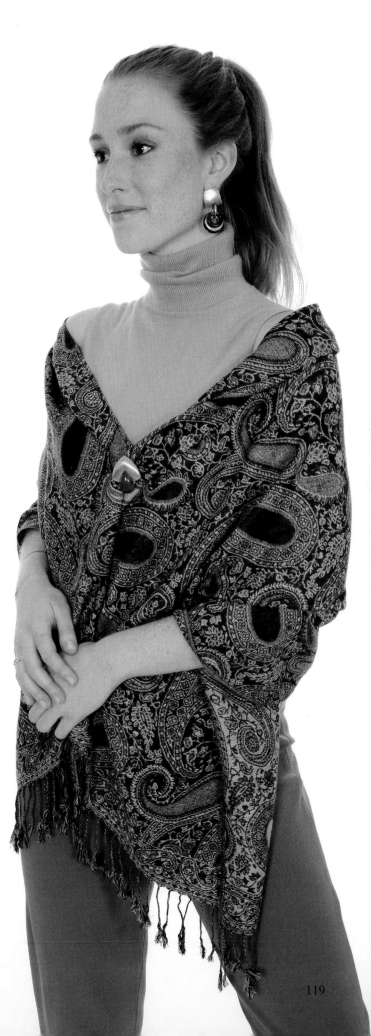

Scarf Ideas

Lots of women tell us they avoid scarves because they aren't sure how to tie them. This versatile favorite works six different ways … and it isn't tied at all.

You'll need:

♦ A rectangular scarf (or large square folded diagonally to a triangle).

♦ A tiny rubber band or a 1/2" plastic curtain ring.

Drape the scarf around your neck with the ends hanging evenly in front. At about bustline level, tuck a little bit of each scarf edge through the rubber band or ring.

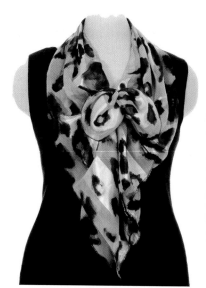

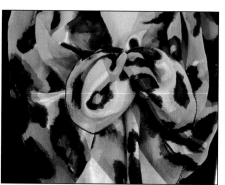

Look #1 — *Gradually pull through more and more fabric to form a mock bow. A close-up is above right.*

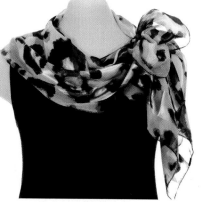

Look #2 — *Rotate the scarf around your neck, bringing the bow to the shoulder. Secure it with a fine safety pin or a bit of double-stick fabric tape.*

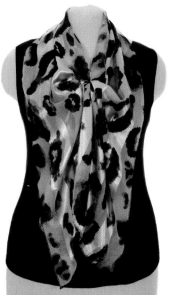

Look #3 — *For variety, use the same technique EXCEPT pull the scarf edges through the ring toward the inside—next to your body. The result is a softly draped jabot.*

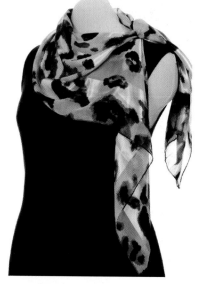

Look #4 — *Rotate the ring to the shoulder, draping one scarf tail to the front and the other to the back.*

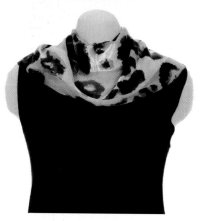

Look #5 — *Rotate the ring to the back. The front forms a graceful cowl. Tuck the tails into the back neckline of your blouse or jacket.*

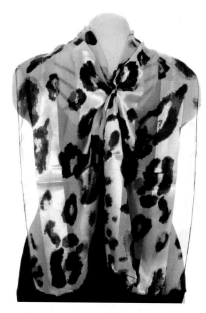

Look #6 — *Or let the tails hang down the back for a romantic look. We call that "exit interest"—style-speak for "somewhere besides your rear end for people to look when you're walking away."*

More Easy Scarf Techniques
For small squares:

Small squares have long been folded diagonally and tied to one side of the neck. Think western movies. Here are some fresh angles on the cowboy scarf!!

Fill an empty neckline or accent a turtleneck or crew sweater with a splash of color. Bring the four corners of a scarf together, right sides in. Poke a finger into the resulting pouch to find the center point. Wrap a tiny rubber band around the fabric over your finger. Remove your finger, flip the scarf back to the right side, concealing the rubber band, and tie two opposite corners behind your neck.

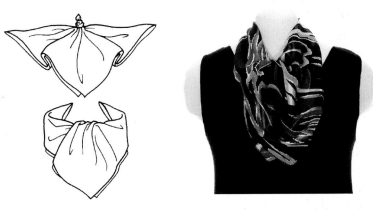

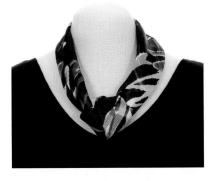

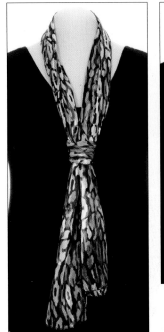

Make a scarf "necklace" with this favorite. Fold two opposite corners to the middle, then roll the new shape into a soft tube. Tie a loose knot at the center of the tube, then knot the free ends behind your neck. Making a tiny knot in back will let the scarf hang in a V shape rather than a choker look if you prefer.

For rectangular scarves:

For all these ties, first fold the scarf softly in thirds lengthwise to control the f

Easiest of all, simply drape the scarf around your neck, with the two sides ha front. Add a jacket to anchor the scarf at the back neckline. This creates a sti line to lengthen and slim your upper body.

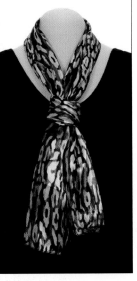

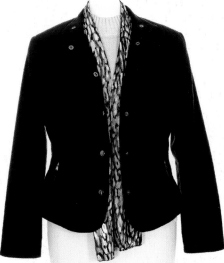

If you prefer to have the scarf secured, simply make a loose overhand knot in one side and slip the remaining end through the knot. (The jacket is now optional, no longer required to hold the scarf in place.) The ends of the scarf should be offset by about 2" to avoid creating a horizontal design line right across your tummy. The position of the knot is also important. Aligned with your bust, it will enhance your visual cup size. Positioned above your bust, it will lift and slightly minimize your bust.

Want this look, but shorter? Hold the two sides of the scarf together, ends offset as above, and tie a single overhand knot through the double layers. Position the knot for the visual effect you prefer.

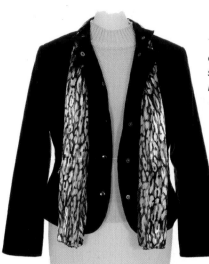

To integrate a blouse or shell color with a contrasting jacket, start with a scarf that incorporates both colors. Fold the jacket collar up slightly at the back of your neck. Drape the scarf around your shoulders behind the collar and forward under the lapels to secure it.

Another series of variations begins with matching the midpoint of the scarf with the center front of your neck, draping the tails over your shoulders to the back. Cross one tail over the other behind your neck and bring each one over its opposite shoulder to the front. Loosen the neckline and leave the tails hanging ...

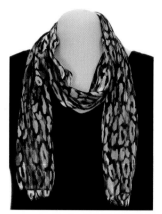

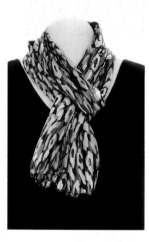

An easy favorite—loop the loop—starts by bringing the two scarf ends together, creating a fold at the midpoint.
Bring the doubled scarf around your neck and tuck the free ends through the loop. What could be easier?

Or drape the tails through the loosened loop once
...or twice

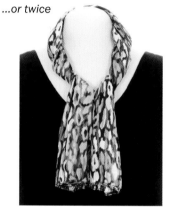

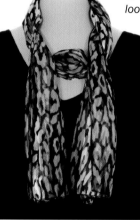

An interesting variation: start the same way, but bring only one free end through the loop. Pull that strand up near your neck and make a figure-8 twist in the loop. Bring the remaining end through the new loop and pull gently down on both scarf ends to settle the fabric into a lovers' knot.

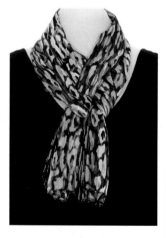

Starting from the original drape (unwrapped), bring one tail over the other, then up through the loop back to front to form an ascot

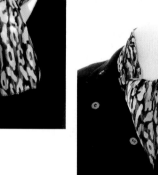

To flatter a shorter or fuller neck, try this loop variation: Start with the two ends together, fold at the midpoint. Put a finger through the middle fold and twirl it to twist the layers tightly together. Bring the resulting twist around your neck, work the ends through the loop and fluff the tails.

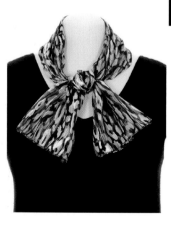

Or, with one tail through the loop, tie both ends into a perky square knot and fluff the loose ends.

To see videos of all these scarf tying techniques, visit NancyNixRice.com/scarfties.html

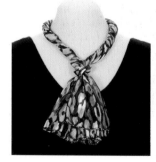

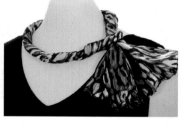

A Large Square Scarf as a Mock Blouse

A large square scarf can even double as a mock blouse. Fold a large square diagonally and tie the upper two corners behind your neck and the two lower corners around your waist, rolling the lower folded edge under as needed to rest at your waist under a jacket.

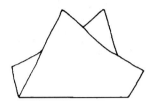

Fold diagonally.

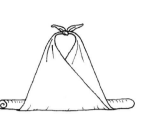

Roll the bottom of scarf up and inward to your waist length and then tie ends behind back.

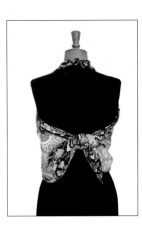

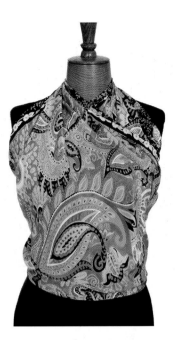

Or Wear a Large Square as a Cocoon Jacket

Need a dressy wrap in a hurry? Choose a large square scarf that complements your outfit and secure the two pairs of adjacent corners with tiny square knots. Slip your arms through the two "sleeves" formed by the knots and presto! —a jacket. Best of all, the back of the faux jacket showcases the beautiful center motif that a large scarf typically features.

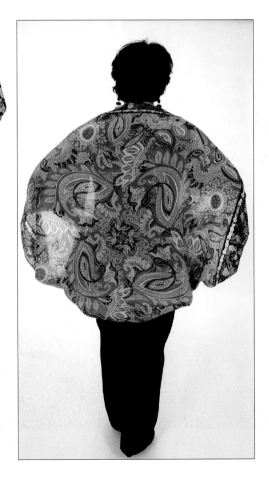

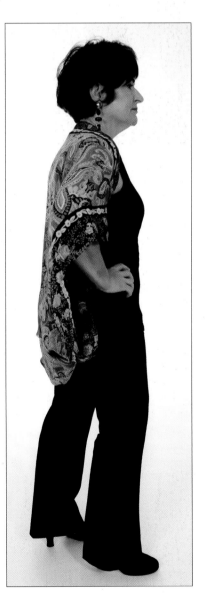

123

Infinity Scarf

An infinity scarf is essentially a tube of fabric. If the tube is wide, begin by folding it in half widthwise, creating a double-layer of fabric half the original width. If you like, fold again, creating a tube that is narrower yet. Drape the tube around your neck, hanging to the front.

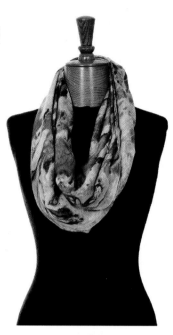

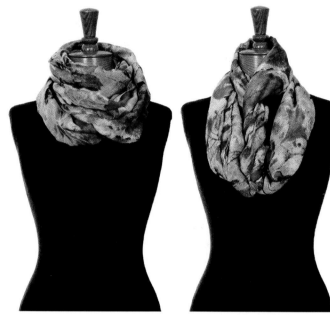

Make a simple figure-8 twist in the hanging portion and bring it over your head to the back of your neck.

Or bring the loop a third time around your neck for a shorter, fuller wrap.

From the same starting position you can also twist the front loop 3-4 times and bring the remaining loop over your head to create a flatter and more controlled look.

Or begin a new technique by folding the loop of fabric in half lengthwise and wrap it behind your neck, with about 1/3 of the length on one side and about 2/3 on the other. Bring the longer end through the loop of the shorter end. Optionally, lift the long end toward your neck and twist the shorter loop end in a figure 8 before bringing the long end back through that new loop.

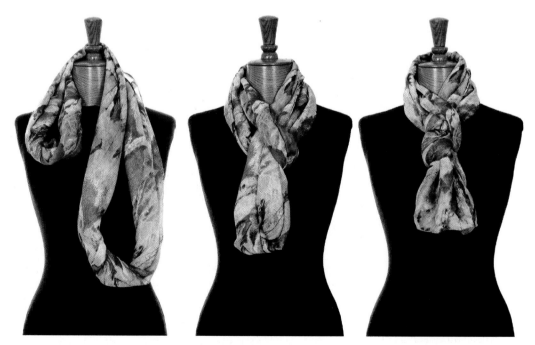

Wearing a Pashmina

These oversized, lightweight shawls come in solids or in tapestry patterns and are surprisingly comfy and easy to wear despite their dramatic presence. A true pashmina is made from the hair of a rare mountain goat and is quite expensive. Wool and silk blends are budget-friendly alternatives. Cheaper polyester and rayon copies look similar but lack the softness and drape, and have a tendency to pill.

Beyond fashion, pashminas have practical applications for warmth. One of our clients keeps several solid color ones in zip-top plastic bags in her car, readily available when she encounters a chilly restaurant or movie theater. And they are a great alternative to a shared airline blanket when you're traveling. Here are some options for wearing one:

Simply toss over your shoulder.

Fold in half lengthwise and pull ends through the loop.

Wear backwards over your shoulders.

Wrapped around your body, slightly off the shoulders and held at center front with a coordinating fashion pin.

Wear off the shoulders and use hands to hold in place or hold in bend of your elbow.

Jewelry Tips and Ideas

Jewelry is the accessory element with the greatest potential for creativity and self-expression. It can add polish to any ensemble, create focal points far from figure challenges, link unexpected color combinations, and take an outfit up or down the formality scale. Jewelry choices fall into three basic categories:

Fine Jewelry – Precious metals and gemstones have timeless appeal, but few of us can afford an extensive wardrobe of statement fashion pieces in this price category.

Bridge Jewelry – Items made from semiprecious stones, shell, enamels and porcelains give a lasting quality look at affordable prices. This category usually offers the best investment for your jewelry wardrobe. The natural materials in fine and bridge jewelry have the added plus of adapting to the colors around them, to blend with a wider range of garments than their cheaper plastic counterparts.

Fashion Jewelry – Budget-friendly fakes can work with very casual looks. These can offer an economical way to adopt the newest fad looks, but seldom add long-term value to your wardrobe.

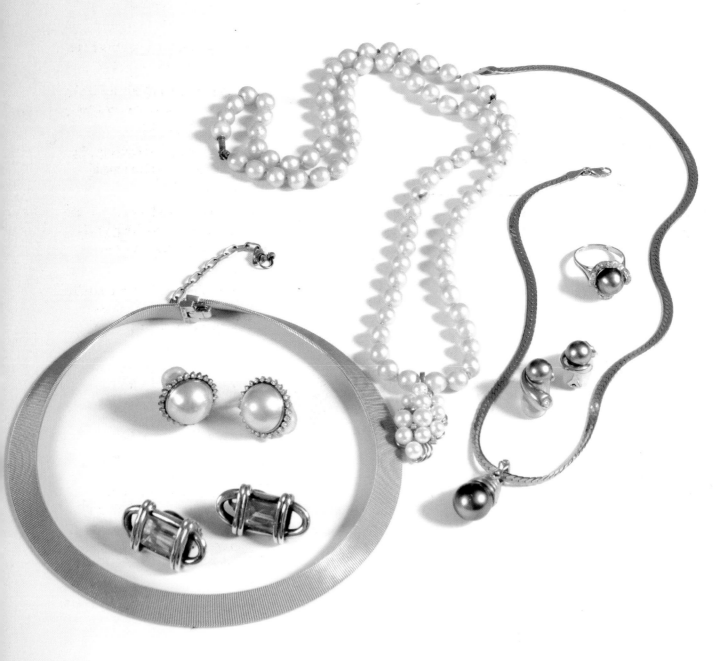

Choose Jewelry Purchases Wisely

It's easy to buy jewelry based solely on its intrinsic loveliness. You'll make better choices when you keep in mind your points of connection.

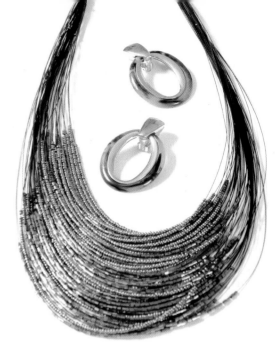

♦ **Color** – Use your color fan as a guide to the metals and stones that will flatter you and work with many items in your wardrobe.

♦ **Body scale** – Larger jewelry items look great on larger bodies, while delicate items would look insignificant. Those same large items would overpower a smaller body frame.

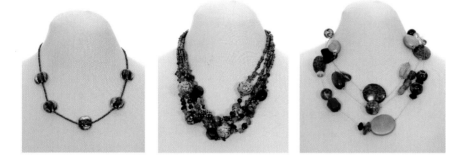

♦ **Facial scale** – If your features are a different scale than your body, jewelry items should connect with both. For example, a bold necklace made up of smaller components would flatter a bold-scale woman with smaller features.

♦ **Facial structure** – The shapes in your jewelry should echo the degree of curve or angularity seen in your facial features.

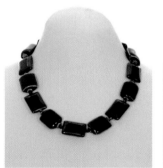 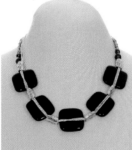 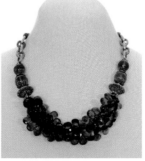

angular   *intermediate*   *curved*

♦ **Which metal?** – Remember the gold/silver test on page 13?

- If one metal looked decidedly better on you, it is your best choice for jewelry.

- If both metals looked equally good, choose mixed metal jewelry.

- If silver looked better, you can still look fine wearing gold in small amounts or in a mix with silver.

- If gold looked better, consider experimenting with brass, copper and tri-tone mixes.

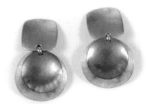

- Rose gold—a mix of gold with copper—has a pinkish cast that is flattering to nearly every woman's coloring.

- ♦ **Personal style** – A woman with a relaxed, casual attitude and lifestyle would look out of harmony wearing an item of very dramatic jewelry or delicate, romantic pieces.

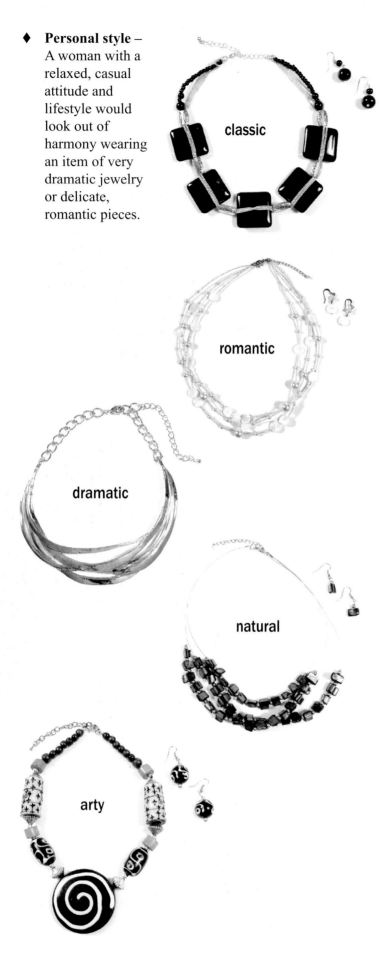

classic

romantic

dramatic

natural

arty

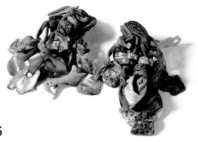

Earrings

Earrings are especially important because of their ability to focus attention toward the face and to add presence to even a casual outfit. Yours will be most effective in your wardrobe if you purchase with these guidelines in mind:

- ♦ **Color** – While any choice from your color fan can work for earrings, stones that relate to your eye color can be especially effective. They make your eyes more prominent, enhancing eye contact and one-on-one communication. Abalone shell has that effect with blue or blue-green eyes. Amber, carnelian and tiger eye emphasize golden brown eyes. Unakite and green agate are lovely with green eyes.

- ♦ **Best metals** – Your best metal options can be personalized even more to make earring choices most effective. For bright, high-contrast coloring, a shiny or faceted metal surface is most flattering. For more gentle, muted coloring, a brushed or burnished finish is a better balance. For women with salt-and-pepper or highlighted brown hair, the darkened lines of an antiqued-finish silver or gold echo that variegated color characteristic.

- ♦ **Body scale** – Coins are one easy guideline—though certainly not a rule—for earring size. If your body scale is small, your most balanced earring size approximates a dime. Medium to large body scale balances easily with nickel or quarter-sized earrings. Grand body scale is proportional with quarter-sized or larger earrings.

- ♦ **Facial proportions** – A wider face is flattered by earrings that are longer than they are wide; they slim and elongate the face. A narrow face looks better with earrings that are a bit wider than their length.

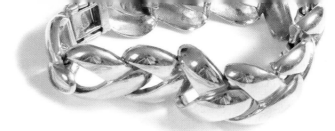

- ◆ **Facial structure** – The degree of curve or angle in an earring design should harmonize with the curve or angularity of your facial features.

- ◆ **Hairstyle** – Longer hairstyles often tend to conceal earrings, requiring a bolder style and scale to make a visual impact. Short haircuts obviously make earrings much more visible.

Here are some examples for different combinations of these factors:

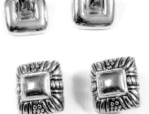

A woman with a wide face and curved features might choose one of these oval earrings—longer than wide, but softly curved.

A woman with a narrow face and more angular features would look good in one of these choices—wider than long and square or rectangular shapes.

A woman with balanced facial proportions and moderately angular features might choose either a square shape softened with three-dimensional styling or a curved shape sharpened by straight-line detail.

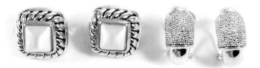

Many women with pierced ears overlook the fact that they can also wear clip-on styles. Clips offer the advantage of varying the placement on your earlobe to create the most flattering proportions with your face. Larger earrings are often more comfortable when their weight is supported by a clip rather than a wire or post. The degree of tension on an earring clip can be adjusted for comfort using a tiny tool called a tension key, widely available online.

Bracelets

Bracelets are a fun and easy way to highlight trim wrists and lovely hands. But remember that most of the time, with arms at your sides, those bracelets end up right next to hips and thighs—areas many women don't particularly want to spotlight.

Minimize that concern by seeking out bracelets that are either oval-shaped to fit closely around the wrist or segmented (links, for example) so they drape slightly. Consider avoiding thick round bangles that stand away from the wrist and add visual bulk to the hip area.

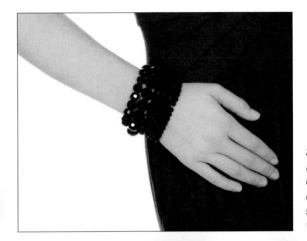

Strands of beads or link chain bracelets conform to the shape of your wrist.

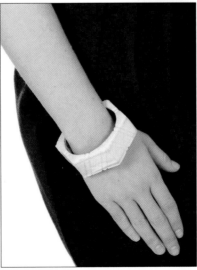

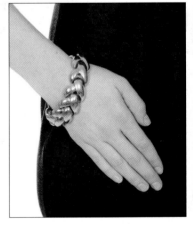

Bangles retain their own shape, potentially adding unwanted visual bulk to your hips.

A favorite charm bracelet style can do double-duty as a necklace when you add a 6" chain extender. See page 131. Conversely, a necklace in the 14-16" range can triple-wrap your wrist and become a bracelet.

Use your creativity to find multiple ways to use jewelry and other accessories.

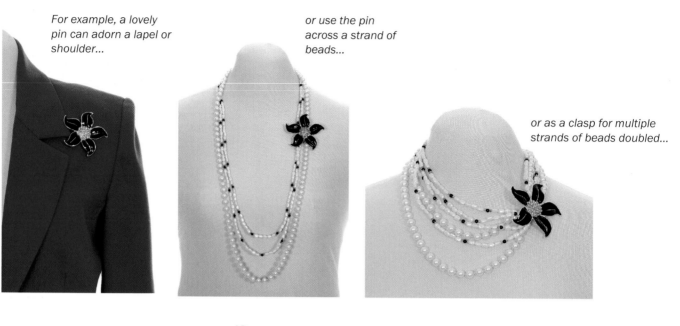

For example, a lovely pin can adorn a lapel or shoulder...

or use the pin across a strand of beads...

or as a clasp for multiple strands of beads doubled...

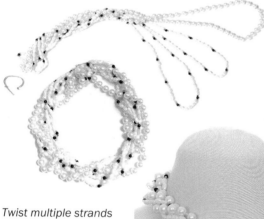

Twist multiple strands together and use a clip to secure strands around the neck. Twisting action compensates for minor differences in lengths of strands.

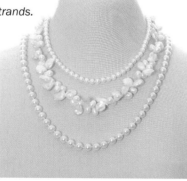

Layer several related strands, spaced at approximately 2" intervals.

Double-wrap a longer strand of beads...

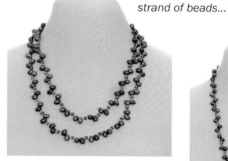

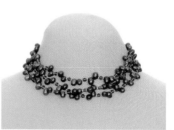

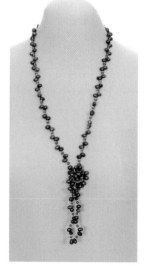

or triple-wrap for greater impact...

or wear full-length and knotted...

Adapt a necklace length to various garment necklines:

Fasten the necklace in the first loop of a chain for the shortest profile.

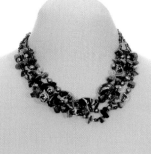

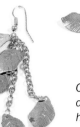

Convert a long, dangle earring by hooking links of the chain over the ear wire.

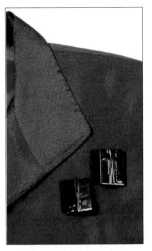

Fasten the necklace in the last loop of a built-in extender for a longer look.

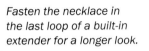

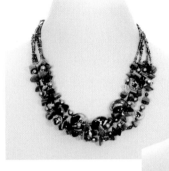

Glue pin-backs to over-sized earrings with clips removed, or poke large pierced earings through the fabric

Add a separate extender chain for 6" of added length.

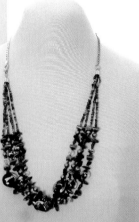

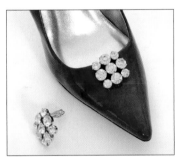

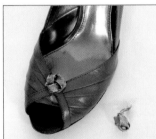

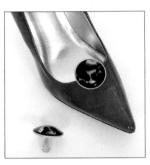

Use a 6" chain extender to make a necklace from a favorite charm bracelet.

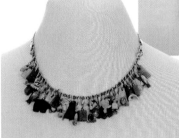

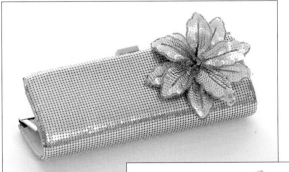

Add a clip earring to a plain pump for an updated look.

Embellish a purse with a colorful scarf.

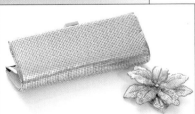

Decorate an evening bag with a jeweled flower pin.

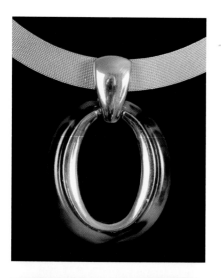

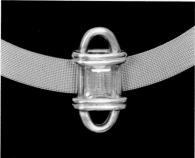

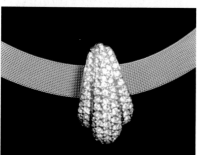

Accessory Capsules

You'll be more likely to have the right accessories for every outfit and occasion if you build your collection in related groupings like the ones pictured here.

Build your first grouping in your key neutral—usually a variation of your hair color. In this important color you'll probably want both a dressy and casual shoe and perhaps a boot. A dressier handbag and a casual one, a wider and a narrower belt and at least one coordinating necklace and earring could round out the basic selection. Scarves that blend your key neutral with fashion accent colors are fun, versatile add-ons.

The shades of your neutral in the grouping should harmonize, but need not be overly matchy-matchy. In fact, some variation gives a more sophisticated look to the outfits you accessorize with these pieces.

Additional accessory capsules might include one in your secondary neutral, one in a fun "pop" color, and one in more casual styles and materials for your casual summer clothes.

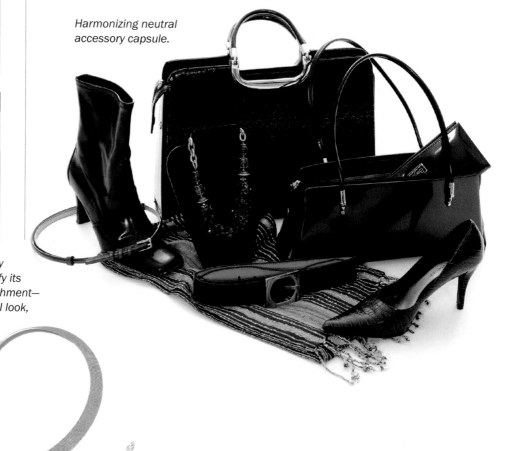

Harmonizing neutral accessory capsule.

This classic gold choker will find its way into many more outfits when you modify its mood by adding a clip earring embellishment—tortoise shell and gold oval for a casual look, amber for a more tailored feeling, or glitzy for after-five wear.

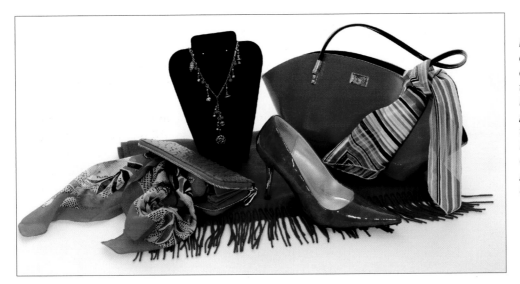

In this accent color collection, one scarf ties the red pieces back to black garments while the other scarf links red to clothing in gray, taupe, and brown.

The variegated colors in the scarf and the pearl necklace allow this accessory capsule to work with a variety of gray shades.

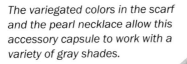

A straw hat, hemp wedge sandal, shell jewelry and sunglasses form the foundation of a summer accessory capsule.

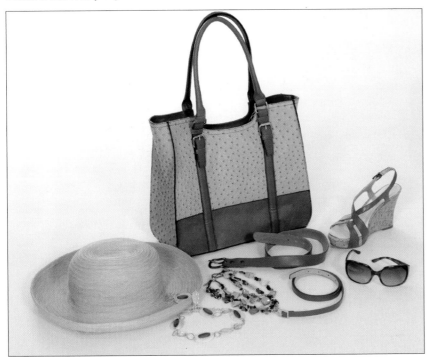

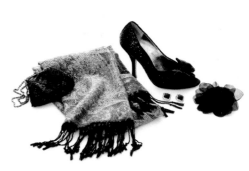

You'll also find accessory capsules to go with your formal capsule on page 107.

Change the Mood of an Outfit With Accessories

Accessories have amazing capacity to shift the look of basic garments for a variety of situations.

Jenny's wool crepe dress is acessorized four ways.

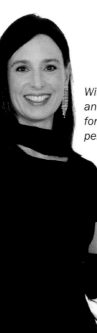

With a lacy shawl, glitzy earrings, and silk and rhinestone pumps for a cocktail event or symphony performance.

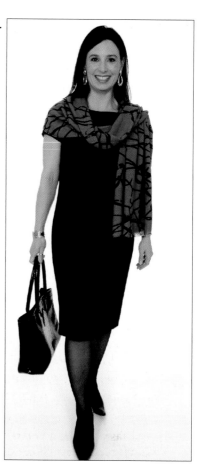

Two casual looks—adding a sweater under the dress and over it (which makes the dress look like a skirt). Black is Jenny's key neutral, but you can create comparable versatility with basic garments in any neutral that flatters you.

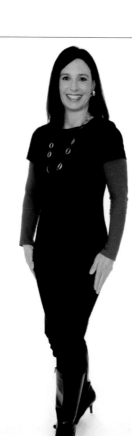

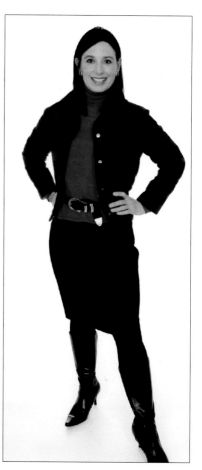

Invisible Accessories

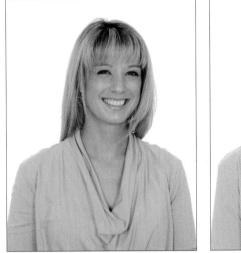
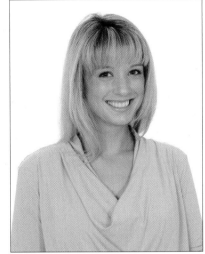

Although they are meant to remain unseen, two accessory items can do wonders to make most women appear taller, trimmer, and better proportioned.

♦ **Shoulder shapes.** Even if you cut the pads out of your washable garments because they clump up in the laundry, you'll almost certainly want to replace them with removable foam ones. The curved shapes fit right over your natural shoulder, and the unglazed surface adheres to the fabric inside the garment. The subtle added lift they provide balances all sorts of fullness lower on your body—hips, thighs, tummy, bust, upper arm—you name it. Wear them in any unstructured jackets, shirts, shells, sweaters and twin sets. They have the added advantage of coming out when you wear the same shirt or shell under a lined jacket with pads of its own built in.

Some women are concerned that shoulder pads are out of fashion at a given moment. Fashion trends refer to the current shoulder line in tailored jackets and its degree of added width. The shoulder shapes we're talking about are an issue of figure balancing, not fashion trends.

Other women fear they'll "look like a fullback" wearing shoulder shapes. Shoulder shapes are much more subtle than that, but if you think about it, football players do appear to have trim hips because their padding provides counterbalance!

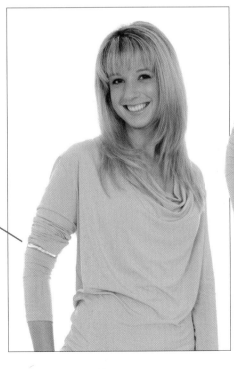

♦ **Sleeve bands.**
Many women feel more comfortable with sleeves pushed up. Others appreciate the lifting, slimming visual effect that pushing up gives an outfit. And nearly all of those women are frustrated when those sleeves keep falling back down.

Sleeve bands are stretchy metal circles that fit like garters just above the elbow, hiding in the folds of fabric and keeping sleeves securely and comfortably pushed up all day.

Dressing Ten Pounds Thinner

A perfectly good garment can still be all wrong ... without the right accessories and details.
Marty salvaged this two-piece knit by making it look much more flattering and you can use these tips too.

- ♦ Balance lower body fullness with subtle shoulder pads.

- ♦ Draw hemline into a flattering diagonal with a buckle.

- ♦ Keep sleeves pushed up with sleeve bands.

- ♦ Shorten skirt to below-knee length.

- ♦ Taper skirt side seams to remove excess width.

- ♦ Add low-vamp pumps or color-toned hose to elongate legs.

- ♦ Brighten makeup and add statement earrings for upward focus.

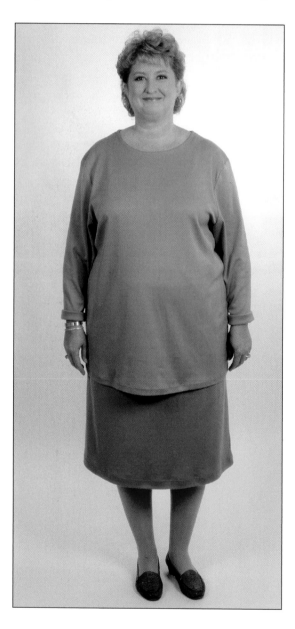
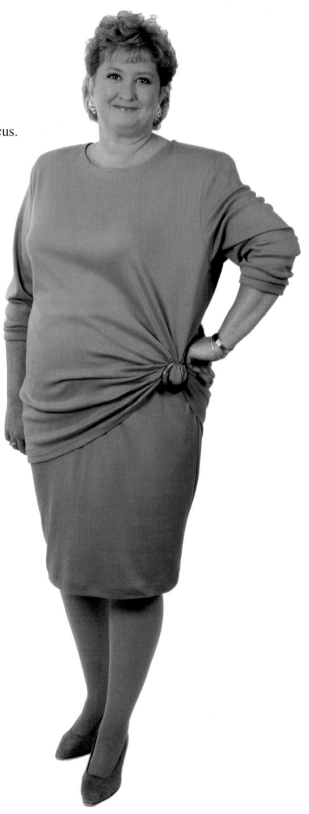

Your Mirror Is Your Most Important Accessory

You may have noticed that recommendations throughout this book are phrased as suggestions to try rather than absolute rules. That's because each woman is a multifaceted combination of traits, and even a seemingly fail-safe recommendation for one of those traits may be overruled by what flatters another.

The solution? Make a full-length mirror your new best friend and key fashion accessory. That's what Emmy did in experimenting with hemlines for her pink cowl-neck top.

The standard guideline suggests avoiding a horizontal hemline at a wider spot on your body—in this case Emmy's hips. She tried varying the look by ruching up some of the length to create a shorter length and slightly curved hem. She also experimented with pulling up just one side to create a diagonal hem.

But because her silhouette dips noticeably inward just above her fullest part, those alternative hemlines expose more than they camouflage. And the supposedly unflattering straight hemline fills out that indentation and is the most flattering option with these body-conscious leggings.

With a skirt or a more body-skimming pant, the ruched or diagonal hemline might indeed be the best choice. She'll know for sure when she follows:

The One Absolute Rule: Always Check Your Mirror.

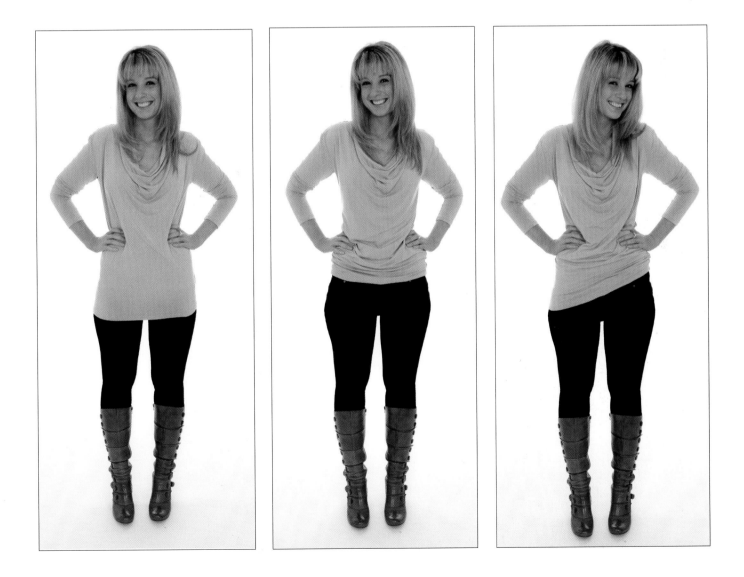

Accessory Add-Up

Wardrobe consultants often teach clients a point system to ensure that a look is neither overdone nor boring. Give yourself one point for each of the following … and an extra point for an item that is exceptionally bold or ornate:

__ **Each visible item of clothing**

__ **Each accent color**

__ **Each patterned/ textured fabric**

__ **Each decorative trim detail**

__ **Each piece of jewelry**

__ **Colored nail polish**

__ **Colored or textured hose**

__ **Handbag**

__ **Briefcase**

__ **Contrast belt**

__ **Scarf**

__ **Decorative buttons**

__ **Eyeglasses**

__ **Low-heeled (not flats) or higher shoes**

__ **TOTAL**

If your total falls below eight you probably need to add an accent or two to avoid looking bland.

If your total is over 14, like our woman shown here, you are probably overdressed. Remove or change something to tone the look down a notch or two.

ALWAYS check your total look

Check yourself front and back in a full-length mirror before leaving the house. Far better to catch a problem yourself than for others to see it all day. (For guidance in fixing common troublemakers, see the chart on page 65.)

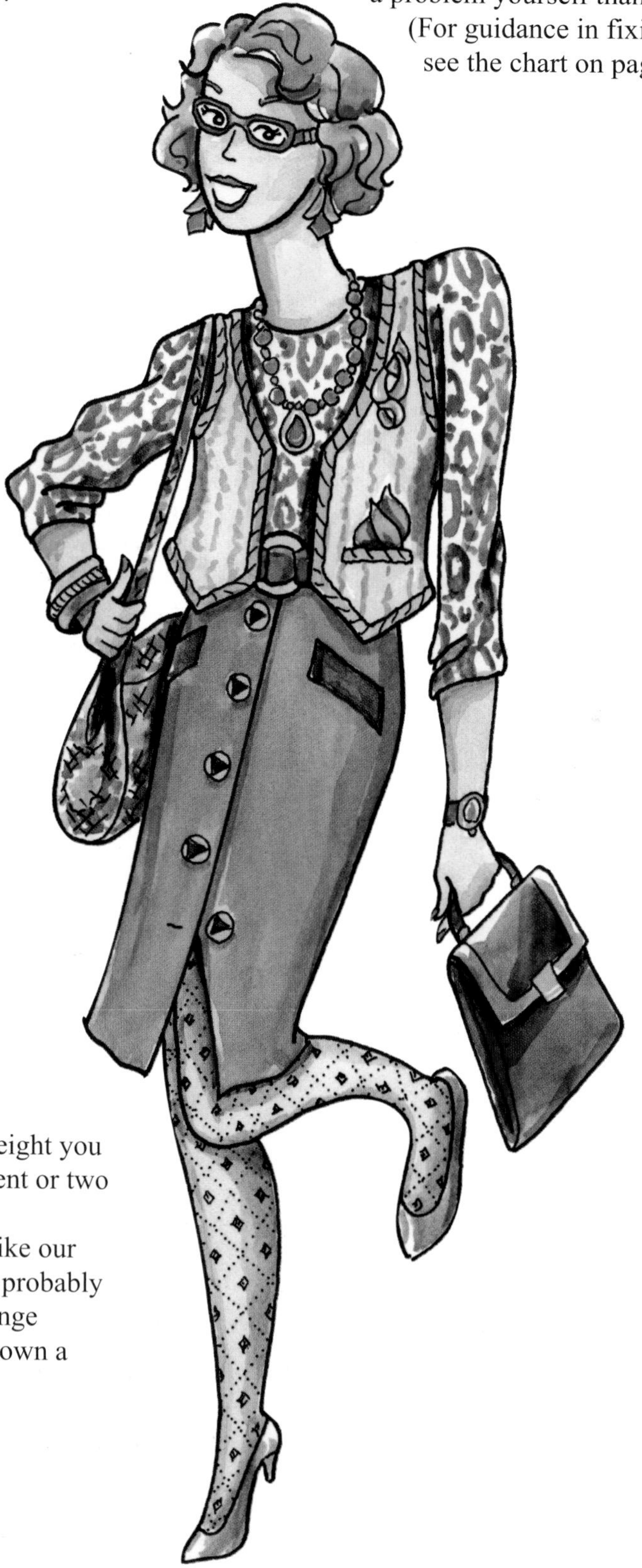

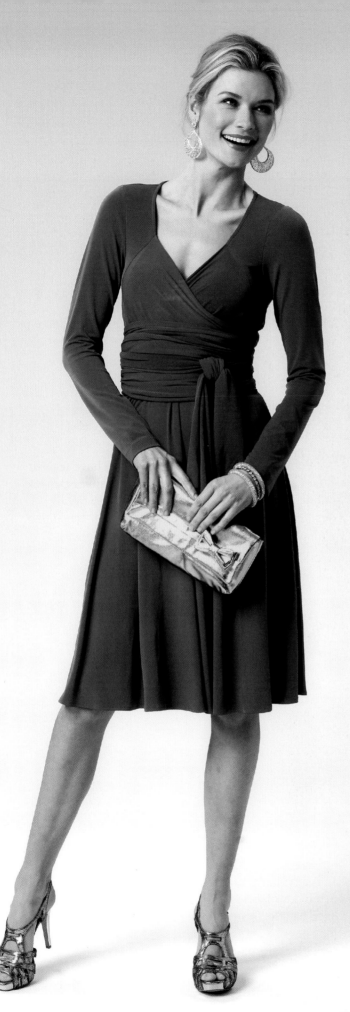

Chapter 13
Undercover Story

No outfit can look better than the body that's wearing it. Fortunately, we can smooth and solidify what Mother Nature (and Ronald McDonald) gave us, thanks to fitting professionals and new techno underlayers.

Bras

Because bra fit is more exacting than garment fit, even a slight weight gain, loss or shift can make a big impact on sizing. Experts say that 8 out of 10 women are wearing the wrong bra size.

The most common mistake: a too-large band (the number) and a too-small cup (the letter). When the band is too large it creeps up in back and droops down in front, so it provides almost no support.

When the cup is too small, you get the pillow effect—one shape within the bra and a second little pillow of flesh above the cup.

Measurements can help define your correct size. Start with a snug measurement of your rib cage, below the bust. Add 5, then round down to the nearest even number to determine your most likely band size.

Next measure your full bust and subtract the band size. Each inch of difference equals a cup size (1" difference = A cup, etc.).

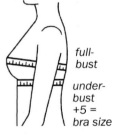

full-bust

under-bust +5 = bra size

up to 1" difference.........	A cup
2" difference	B cup
3" difference	C cup
4" difference	D cup
5" difference	DD

But measurements don't tell the whole story. Like shoes, each bra fits differently, so trying on is a must. Look for styles with the cup design you need.

♦ For firmer (read: younger) tissue, a demi-cup can work just fine.

♦ For softer tissue (from maturity, weight loss, recent pregnancy) a full-coverage cup provides more flattering shape.

- For maximum support, choose underwired styles. In the correct size, you won't even feel the wire. But you'll see the results.

- To appear smaller-busted, choose a minimizer style with a seamless, rounded cup designed to redistribute breast tissue slightly side-to-side and minimize forward projection.

- To look fuller, choose a maximizer style with a seamed cup and good side coverage to push tissue toward the center and increase projection.

- To ramp up cleavage, find a push-up style with padding in the lower half of the cup. (Or you can add removable booster pads to the good bras you already own.)

- To prevent anatomical details from showing through lightweight T-shirts or sweaters, find a style with foam-lined cups (different from a true padded bra that adds volume).

With an assortment of possibilities in the dressing room, try on each one and evaluate for comfort and lift.

To put on a bra correctly, bend from the waist as you slip your arms through the straps, so the breasts "pour" into the cups. Hook the bra below the shoulder blades, then stand upright and adjust the straps.

A properly fitted bra should feel so natural you can forget you have it on. It should close comfortably on the second hook, and it should lift your bust so the fullest point hits halfway between your belly button and that little hollow at the base of your neck. The higher your bust, the longer your torso appears and the slimmer you look.

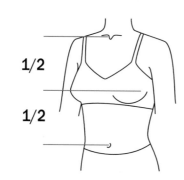

For the final test, slip a body-skimming lightweight T-shirt on over the bra. Its outline will immediately spotlight fit problems you might miss focusing on the bra alone.

Choose a bra—and other undergarments too— in a color near your skin tone to minimize shadowing through lightweight or light-colored clothing. Black is a good alternative under opaque dark garments; white is often too bright and shows through.

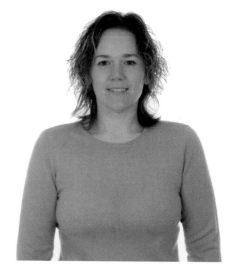

Cindy's white bra underneath shows through; a nude-color one would not.

Perfect bra fit is an art. Some stores have trained fitters on staff, but many do not. Alternatively, check online for a lingerie specialty store, or ask your department store when they have an event scheduled with a fitting expert from one of their suppliers.

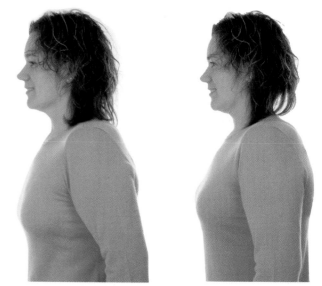

Cindy before a bra fitting.   *After—a subtle flattering lift.*

Bra lines (and panty lines, too) are becoming less an issue thanks to "vanishing edge" designs that use firmly knit fabric requiring no elastic finish. Wider back panels, front closures and front strap adjustment further minimize any visible evidence of the bra under soft, drapable garments.

Panties

Cotton granny-panties have given way to an assortment of briefs (and briefer) with sleeker profiles.

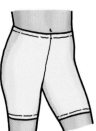

- **Slipshorts** provide maximum coverage. The longer length smooths the silhouette and prevents panty lines.

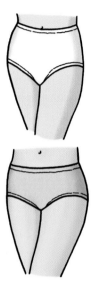

- **Traditional briefs** ride just below the waist and end at the leg joint, just outside the panty-line range on most bodies and under most fabrics.

- **Modern briefs** feature a low waist, ideal under low-rise pants.

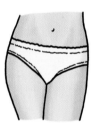

- **Bikini** styles sit 3"-4" below the waist and have a higher leg cut. Cute, but at the risk of showing slight indentation in soft tissue.

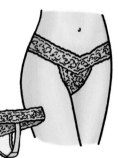

- **Thong** undies have a triangle-shaped front panel, narrow sides and minimal coverage in back, making them practically panty-line-proof. Some women find them incredibly comfortable, others find them utterly unappealing. Our advice—don't knock it if you haven't tried it.

Breathability is important in panties, but newer microfibers and mesh fabrics work as well as cotton and have a smoother look under sleek clothing.

Once you find the style and size you love, it makes sense to watch for seasonal specials and stock up for the year.

Hosiery

Body shaping panty hose do wonders for smoothing tummy, hips and thighs. And they can eliminate visible panty lines. These shaping nylons differ from older control-top styles because the percentage of spandex diminishes gradually from waist to toes rather than ending abruptly in the middle of the thigh, which created an unattractive and uncomfortable bulge.

Because of their compacting effect, consider buying one size larger than your height/weight dimensions indicate to prevent a bulge of tissue above the waist.

Camisoles

Once just a modesty layer, today camisoles now come in spandex-blend fabrics that smooth the soft tissue through your torso. They also control any hint of bulge above the top of your shaper panty hose. They are available in various degrees of control; pick the one that creates the right balance of smoothing and comfort for all-day wear.

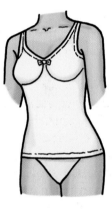

To avoid flattening your bustline too, look for styles that end under the bust, are heat-shaped to accommodate your curves, or incorporate a foam-cup or underwire bra right into the camisole. Tuck the lower edge into your panties or panty hose to avoid a visible ridge.

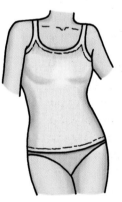

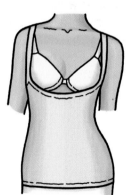

Power Shapers

Call them shapewear, body shapers, slimmers—whatever—but put on one of these techno under layers and you'll look instantly trimmer and more sleek. Choose from these categories:

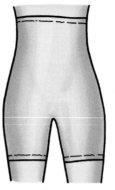

♦ **Tummy/thigh shapers** are body-compressing shorts that end just above or below the knee—not at a soft spot where the garment edge could create a bulge. The upper edge might ride at your waistline or extend all the way up to the bottom of your bra. Look for styles with extra hold at your personal trouble spots.

tummy/thigh shaper

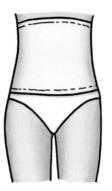

♦ **Waist shapers** extend from just under your bust to your hip bone to minimize waist width.

waist shaper

♦ **Slip shapers** typically include a built-in bra and a slip layer over a snap-crotch panty—ideal under silky dresses.

When you shop for these wonder garments, consider that not all shapers are created equal. Even within a category, each brand or style has a particular emphasis. Some excel at making the tummy flatter; others do miracles for the butt and thigh area. Choose the shaper that's created for the specific advantages you want.

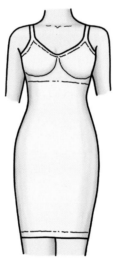

slip shaper

A shaper should be so comfortable you forget you're wearing it. If it's uncomfortable you'll leave it in the drawer … and it won't do your figure any favors in there. Pick the item that corrects your specific issue—tummy, hips, thighs—and nothing more.

Despite the tendency to buy the smaller size in order to get more squoosh value, you should actually do the opposite. If you're packed too tightly, the result will inevitably be bulges instead of a smooth line. Try on the actual item to determine your most flattering fit. This is one time you don't want to order online.

Price correlates to both the number of body areas impacted and the quality of the fabric and construction. Don't pay for features you don't need, but do pay for the best quality you can afford. The best-known shaper brands are fairly pricey. Some of the same companies make more affordable lines that are not quite as powerful or as beautifully finished and are sold through discount retailers.

Lingerie Care

Wash undergarments by hand or in a cool-water gentle machine cycle. Use Ivory soap or a specialty lingerie cleaner. Avoid Woolite, which is formulated for natural fibers, not synthetics. Heat breaks down spandex fibers, so skip the dryer and line dry instead.

Chapter 14
About Face

Style doesn't just happen from the neck down. Your choices in makeup, hair color and style, and eyeglasses can make or break your total look. Once again, the secret to great choices is maximizing points of connection.

Mastering Makeup

Even the most spectacular wardrobe can't create your best appearance if your face is either unfinished or overdone.

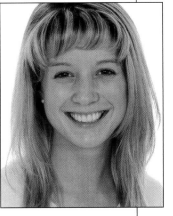

Far too many women skip makeup entirely because they want a natural look. But the truth is that well-done makeup actually looks more natural than your bare face.

Your color fan is the best guide for choosing makeup colors that will enhance your own coloring in a soft, natural way.

♦ Foundation should match your skin tone as exactly as possible.

♦ Eye shadow colors should include:
  • A base color that blends with your skin tone
  • An accent color that relates to your hair color.
  • A second accent that either repeats or complements your eye color.

♦ Blush and lip colors should blend with the reds from your fan. The red color family includes everything from pinks and peaches, through mid-value corals and reds, to darker rusts and wine shades. Most women like to have at least three lipsticks and nail colors— the palest, mid and darker versions from their particular color range.

♦ Eyeliner and mascara relate to your color temperature and value. Cool women can choose dark brown, charcoal gray or navy; warm women look best in variations of warm brown. Few women look natural wearing black liner or mascara.

When you choose makeup colors this way, they will blend with everything in your wardrobe. You won't need special makeup colors for each outfit. How beautifully simple!

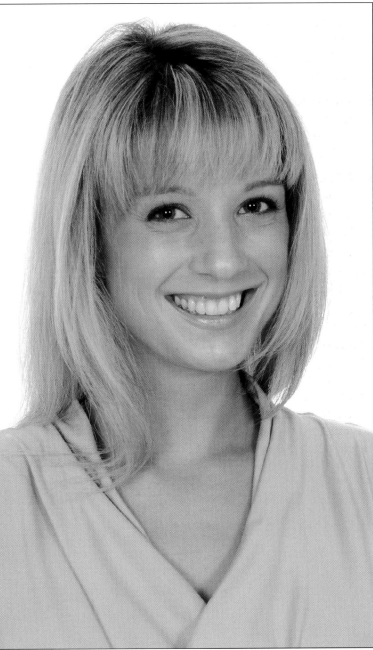

The 10-Minute Face

Styles in makeup application change over time, but with these instructions you can complete a timeless, classic look in less than 10 minutes.

Use the grid below to apply samples of your color to the face, recording their names in the boxes at the right. See page 146 for examples.

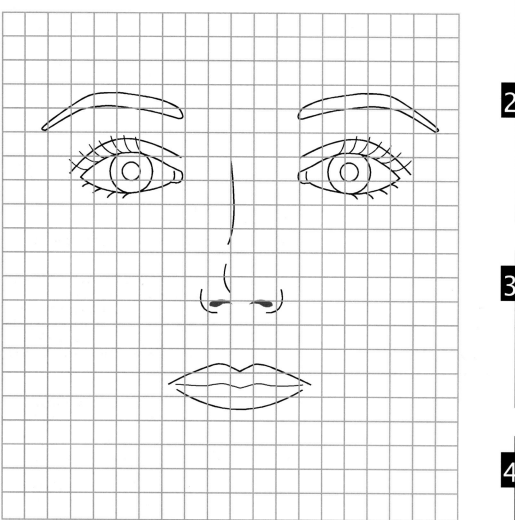

Evaluate your finished makeup application in a full-length mirror as part of your head-to-toe look. You should see your features more distinctly, but barely notice the makeup itself.

Don't be surprised if your first trial of our "10-Minute Face" takes a little longer. With a few days of practice you'll soon reach an efficient pace.

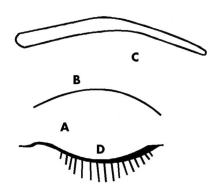

1. Color-correction cream colors:
_____
_____
_____

2. Foundation color:
_____
_____

3. Shadow concealer color:
_____

4. Powder color:
_____

5. Eye shadow colors:
A. _____
B. _____
C. _____
Eyeliner color:
D. _____

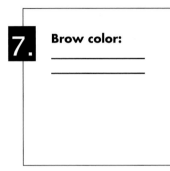

6. **Mascara colors:**

brown _____
navy _____
black _____

7. **Brow color:**

_____
_____

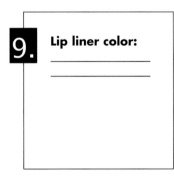

8. **Blush color(s):**

softer_____
deeper_____
_____

9. **Lip liner color:**

_____
_____

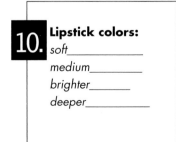

10. **Lipstick colors:**

soft_____
medium_____
brighter_____
deeper_____

Step 1: Conceal any unwanted coloration with a correction cream.

These use basic color theory to neutralize a color by blending with its complement:

♦ Conceal redness with mint green.

♦ Conceal sallowness (yellow) with lilac.

♦ Conceal blue-purple veins with yellow.

Dot the cream on the discolored areas; blend with a makeup sponge until it looks slightly chalky.

Step 2: Even out skin tone with foundation.

Pour a bit of liquid onto a makeup sponge, dot onto face as shown, then blend with downward strokes of the sponge.

Step 3: Conceal dark circles and creases.

Dot concealer with a cotton swab into dark under-eye areas and any creases; blend with sponge.

Step 4: Set these layers with powder.

Brush on a light coating of finely milled loose powder for a velvety look. Try powdering just one side of your face and look at the difference!

Step 5: Emphasize your eyes.

Eye shadow isn't a mystery. First apply a pale shadow (A)—close to your skin color—to the entire lid from lashes to brows. Accent the crease with a horizontal band of deeper neutral (B) just below the brow bone. Add color accent (C) in the outer corner. Blend with a sponge applicator or brush. Finish with a pencil liner along the base of the lashes (from inner edge of the iris to outer corner on top; outer third on the bottom). Blend the pencil with a cotton swab.

Step 6: Define lashes with mascara.

Use the applicator side to side (like a windshield wiper) across lash tips first; follow with lengthwise strokes. Add a second coat for more definition.

(NOTE: Replace mascara every 90 days to avoid bacterial contamination, but rinse and clean the old applicator and use it to comb through mascara'd lashes to separate and de-clump.)

Step 7: Define brows to frame your eyes.

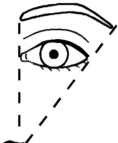

Fill in any gaps with a soft pencil or powdered brow color, following your natural shape. Apply a clear brow gel to define and control the shape; brush it through the brows; then style them into a lifted arch. (NOTE: If you tweeze your brows or have them professionally waxed, coat the area first with baby teething gel to numb the "ouch.")

Step 8: Brighten your face with blush.

Use a soft blush brush to apply color from the hairline near the top of the ear toward the center of the face along the cheekbone. This slightly higher placement visually lifts the face and emphasizes the eyes. Use a sponge to blend the edges of the color for a softer, natural look.

Step 9: Enhance your lip shape with liner.

Sketch a line of color outlining the top and bottom lips. Create a fuller look by lining along the ridge of skin where the lip structure begins. Or minimize full lips by lining just inside that ridge, where natural color begins. Add fill-in strokes within the outline and blend with fingertip. Coloring the entire lip avoids a visible outline and maintains color after lipstick wears away.

Step 10: Finish the face with lipstick.

Apply right from the tube or use a brush for more precise application. The matte or glossy finish adds polish to your look while the emollient ingredients keep lips moist and conditioned.

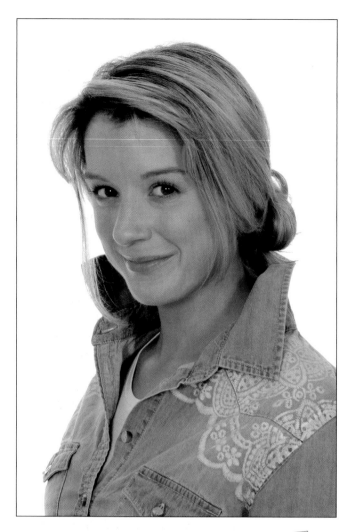

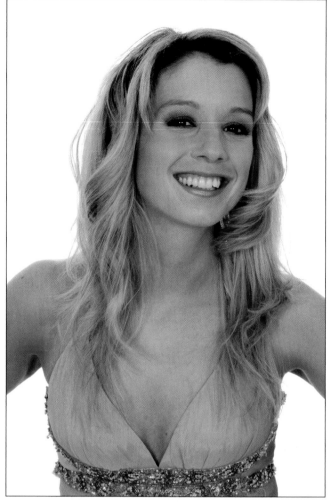

Casual Face

For casual occasions a lighter makeup look is appropriate.

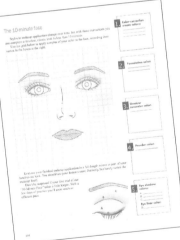

- Apply foundation with a damp sponge for more sheer coverage. Or substitute a tinted moisturizer.
- Skip the accent eye shadow colors; use only base color and pencil liner. Keep mascara light.
- Keep lip colors pale or neutral.
- Use blush generously for a healthy glow.

Glamour Face

For evenings and special occasions, stronger makeup colors and more dramatic applications are ideal.

- Use bolder eye shadow accent colors or apply your usual colors more heavily. Eyeliner is definitely noticeable.
- Brows are more defined and lashes need several coats of mascara.
- Lipstick colors can be more intense and glossy or shimmery.
- Use brighter blush, but in a very sheer application to keep focus on eyes and lips.

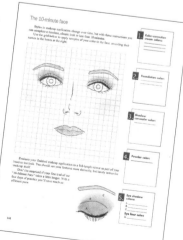

Skin Care Basics

Healthy skin is critical to a good makeup application. A good skin-care program can significantly slow the inevitable aging process.

Lifestyle factors are as important as creams and lotions in caring for the skin. Skin is, after all, a body organ so all the factors that contribute to overall health also help develop glowing skin.

♦ Getting adequate sleep gives skin cells downtime to produce new cell layers.

♦ Drinking six to eight glasses of water daily hydrates the skin from within and flushes away the by-products of cellular reproduction.

♦ Eating a healthful diet provides nutritional building blocks for new tissue growth.

♦ Avoiding caffeine and nicotine prevents constricted (tightened) blood vessels. When blood flows freely it carries nutrients more efficiently to developing skin cells.

♦ Minimizing sun exposure prevents ultraviolet rays from damaging the connective tissue in the skin's supporting layer. Dermatologists call sun exposure the single greatest cause of premature aging and wrinkling.

Understanding how skin grows helps clarify the need for proper skin care. New cells are produced in the innermost layer and are gradually pushed toward the top by even newer cells as they form.

This migration takes about 21 days, and by the time a cell reaches the surface it has lost most of its natural moisture and plumpness. Eventually the surface cells are sloughed off.

The under layer, the dermis, nourishes and supports the outer layer. It contains blood vessels to feed developing cells and elastin and collagen to keep skin firm. It includes sweat glands and sebaceous glands that empty oil and perspiration through the pores.

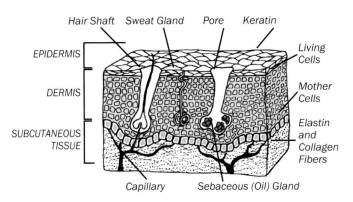

Hair Shaft   Sweat Gland   Pore   Keratin

EPIDERMIS

DERMIS

SUBCUTANEOUS TISSUE

Living Cells

Mother Cells

Elastin and Collagen Fibers

Capillary   Sebaceous (Oil) Gland

Daily Skin Care

Effective skin care can take just moments each morning and evening. It consists of:
♦ Cleansing to remove surface debris and makeup.
♦ Exfoliating to remove dead surface cells.
♦ Moisturizing to keep skin supple.

Regardless of the brand of skin care you choose, it's important to use a compatible group of products. Each line is formulated so the components work together for optimum results. Mixing brands can cause unexpected reactions.

Cleansing

A facial cleanser lifts away makeup, oil, perspiration and pollutants without stripping the skin of moisture or leaving a residue. Apply cleanser to the face with an upward/outward motion and massage gently. Rinse with a soft washcloth and tepid water.

Some skin care systems include a toner to re-establish the skin's normal pH balance. Stroke the liquid over the skin with a cotton ball. Or transfer it to a spray bottle and spritz it on. Other cleansers are themselves pH balanced and don't require a companion toner.

Exfoliating

Exfoliating removes dead cells from the skin's surface so the younger, fresher ones underneath are visible. This can be done manually with a textured product that scrubs away the outer cells. Or it can be done chemically instead. Products containing alpha-hydroxy acids break down the chemical bonds between dead cells, perspiration and body oils so the debris rinses away without scrubbing.

Moisturizing

Moisturizers protect the skin against drying, keep it soft and supple, and minimize wrinkling. A light film of moisturizer in the morning helps makeup go on smoothly and serves as a buffer against pollutants in the air. A richer moisturizer nourishes the skin during its nighttime rejuvenation process. Women with oilier skin need an oil-free moisturizer applied sparingly.

Anti-Aging Products

Although there is no real Fountain of Youth, scientific advances do make it possible to help accelerate the skin's natural renewal process by enhancing collagen production. Visit with a skin care specialist to learn more about which additional products may be right for your situation.

Eyewear

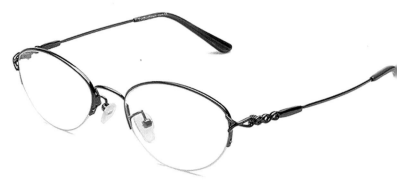

You can make a spectacle of yourself—in the best way—by selecting frames that complement your coloring, facial shape and facial structure.

Gold or tortoise-shell frames look great on women with warm coloring.

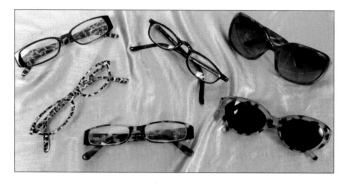

Cool women look better in silvery metals or subtly marbleized blue or wine.

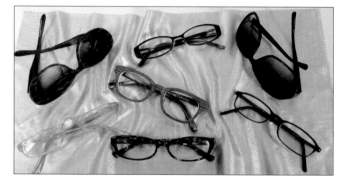

If you have only one pair of glasses, don't opt for bold fashion colors. Frames should enhance your face, not accent your ensemble. If you want to make a color-coordinated fashion statement, invest in an extra pair or two to have fun with. Or buy fun colors in inexpensive readers rather than pricey prescription eyewear.

Although other image books combine facial shape and structure into one concept, you will make much better eyewear choices if you consider the two factors separately. That means determining the horizontal/vertical design of your frames to either narrow a wide face or widen a thin one. Then choose the frame's shape and details to repeat (NOT contrast with) the curve or angularity of your features. See pages 75-76 if you need a refresher about shape and structure.

To narrow a wide face, look for frames with a minimum of strong horizontal emphasis. Rimless frames, clear or pale frames, and frames with a slight upward angle all avoid horizontal focus. Positioning the bridge—the area between the lenses—relatively high, and attaching the side pieces high on the frame also elongate and slim a wide face.

To widen an overly narrow face, choose frames that do have horizontal emphasis. Slightly darker or heavier frames, frames just slightly wider than your face, decorative detail at the outer corners and contrasting side pieces that attach lower on the frame will all add visual width.

The actual shape of the frames should relate to the dominant shape of your features. More squared or rectangular frames enhance angular facial features. Softly curved frames are compatible with curved features. And of course frames with a blend of curves and angles enhance a face with in-between features.

Frames can also emphasize or minimize specific features. For example:

♦ A large nose is minimized by frames with a slightly lower bridge (the area between the lenses).

♦ A higher bridge avoids minimizing an already small nose.

♦ Closely spaced eyes will look more balanced wearing glasses with a clear or lightweight bridge.

♦ A heavier or darker bridge will make wide-spaced eyes appear closer together.

Gear your eye makeup to your glasses. A prescription for farsightedness will magnify the eyes—and the eye makeup. Apply subtle colors with a light touch and balance with brighter lip color. On the other hand, a prescription for nearsightedness will minimize eyes. Counter with bolder eye makeup and slightly softer lip color.

Shopping for Eyeglasses

Anna used these guidelines when she set out to find an updated pair of glasses. She has a playful personality and wanted something fun and different, but also flattering and not too extreme. Below you can see several misses and, finally, a hit.

Very angular frames don't harmonize with Anna's softly curved features.

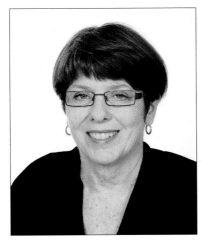

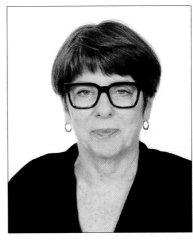

These dark, heavy frames draw attention to the glasses and away from Anna. The high, dark bridge makes her nose look larger too

This oversized style dwarfs her small face, and the frames cover her eyebrows.

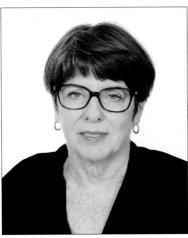

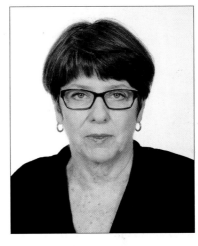

This blue-purple pair clashes with her coloring and gives her a tired look.

This pair comes close. It captures her personality but its extreme roundness doesn't quite blend with her features and it is narrow for her face.

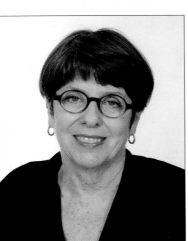

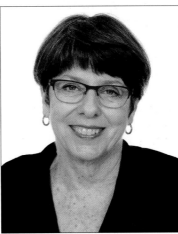

Finally! This pair balances the scale of Anna's face and the gentle curve of her features. The color blends with her hair and brows and the touch of green reflects her playful personality without overpowering her face.

Hair Color

Surveys indicate that between two-thirds and three-quarters of American women color their hair. Here are some tips to ensure that any chemical enhancement you undertake will be flattering and natural looking.

♦ Don't make a radical change from your natural color. One or two shades lighter or darker, in the same hue family, are usually the best choices.

♦ Stay within your color temperature range. Red hair on a cool-skinned person almost always looks artificial, for example. And it constantly surrounds her face with a color she would probably never select in her wardrobe.

♦ For lighter color, but with lower maintenance, try highlighting some strands near your face.

♦ To minimize emerging gray in darker hair, try lowlighting—the same approach as highlights, but creating strands of dark color instead.

♦ Hair color products vary in their coverage, from translucent to opaque. Using a more sheer color lets the natural light/dark variation of your hair show through.

♦ Before you commit to a big change, try out a new color with a wash-out color rinse, a wig, or with an online virtual "makeover."

Warm and cool women often take opposite approaches to coloring as their hair starts to lose pigment. Gray strands sprinkled through warm hair colors typically give the look of very well-done highlights, so warm women tend not to add chemical color in the earlier phases of change. Dark, cool hair, on the other hand, tends to look drab and lifeless with early gray, so these women tend to keep up their original color.

However, as that cool hair becomes more overall gray, it has a lovely silvery quality that many women enjoy showcasing. Fully grayed warm hair often has a dull yellowish cast, so those women may be happier opting for a subtle golden blonde or strawberry blonde color enhancement.

Hairstyle

Hairstyle is a very visible component of your total image … and often a challenging one. Even a recent Miss America credited her title to avoiding a "bad hair day." It's worth a significant investment of time and money to find a stylist who can create the look that's right for:

♦ Balancing your facial shape.

♦ Harmonizing with the curves/angles of your facial structure.

♦ Enhancing your hair's natural texture.

♦ Expressing your personal style.

♦ Using your styling expertise (or lack thereof).

A change in hairstyle can add or diminish fullness in your facial shape, creating the illusion of the fashion-ideal oval.

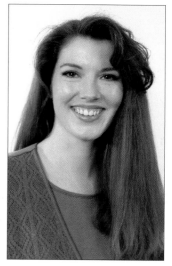

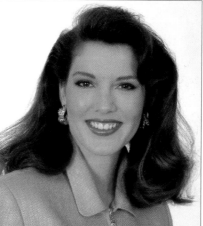

You've already seen these women in Chapter 6, where we talk about face shape, but they perfectly illustrate the point here about hairstyles too.

♦ Fullness at the sides adds width to a narrow face.

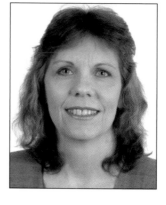

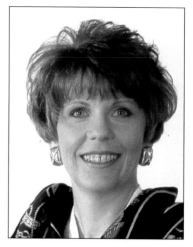

- Sleek sides and pulled-back styles slim a wider face.

- Bangs shorten an overly long face (heavier bangs have more impact than thin or side-swept ones).

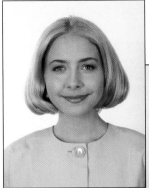

- Hair brushed up off the forehead lengthens a short face.

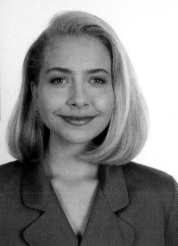

Hairstyle can also move emphasis toward or away from particular facial features.

- A center part draws attention to the nose.

- A side part and side-swept bangs put focus toward the eyes.

Also decide in front of a mirror whether your jaw line and facial features are more angular (think of Cher or Barbra Streisand) or more softly rounded (like Rosie O'Donnell or Oprah Winfrey).

Angular faces look most harmonious with hairstyles, accessories and clothing details that are similarly angular.

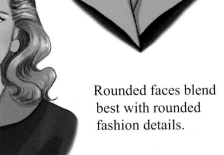

Rounded faces blend best with rounded fashion details.

Texture

Fine hair gains bulk from a blunt cut no more than chin length. Substitute tapering for layering if you want a softer look around the face. Body-building shampoos and setting lotions add volume, but their slight residue means you'll need to shampoo more frequently.

Medium hair is easiest to handle. Blunt cuts create a bulkier, fuller look than angled cuts that make hair lie closer to the head. Layered cuts add fullness.

Coarse hair can look bushy if not carefully shaped. Avoid volume-enhancing blunt cuts. Moderate length adds some control to coarse hair. Or go very short and let it curl. Use a softening conditioner and skip setting lotions.

Be cautious about straightening very curly hair. The harsh chemicals, if overused, can leave hair looking like straw.

Working With Your Stylist

Don't be intimidated to tell even the most celebrated stylist what you want in a haircut. His/her expertise plus your communication can add up to the style of your dreams. The stylist needs to know:

- How much money and time you're willing to spend on maintenance cuts.

- Whether you have the time and expertise for blow drying, special brush techniques, and the like.

- Special demands of your career or lifestyle.

- The kind of clothing you usually wear.

- Any body challenges you want your hairstyle to minimize.

- Past styles you've loved or hated.

Hairstyle Makeovers

Updating the hairstyles made a big difference in the makeovers you see throughout this book. Here are the details about three of them.

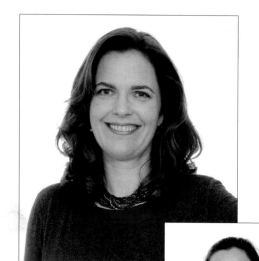

Andrea

Andrea was ready for a new hairstyle, but didn't want to go too short because her naturally curly hair gets unruly without some length to weight 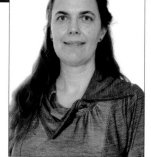 it into place. She had defaulted to just growing it long and pulling it off her face with clips, so there was wonderful potential for an update.

A shoulder-length cut with layers and long, side-swept bangs takes advantage of her curl to create a soft and sophisticated look.

She also wanted a color update to cover a hint of gray and conceal the remnants of a prior red dye job. The stylist used her natural brown color and a hint of reddish-brown as highlights and lowlights to give her hair a lift. The variegated color helps showcase the curves in her hair too.

Now Andrea looks like the successful career woman she is.

Jane

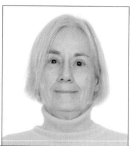

Jane felt that her appearance had gotten drab and that people no longer thought of her as the energetic, enthusiastic, creative person she really is. Her silvery white hair is too striking to even consider coloring. But its texture is very fine and thin, so a layered cut adds body and the appearance 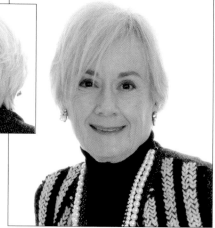 of volume. The spikey, angular bangs add some edge to the look while they minimize her long forehead and bring attention to her eyes.

Stronger makeup colors bring her features into clear focus, and the statement earrings anchor the entire transformation. The new look makes it easy to see her spunky, vibrant personality.

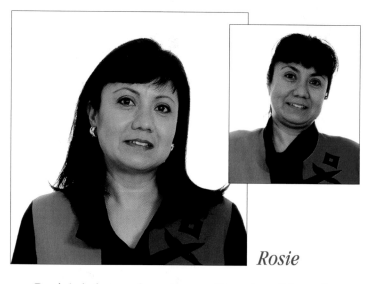

Rosie

Rosie's hair transformation—although striking—is unbelievably simple. It isn't a new color or even a new cut. We simply restyled it in an asymmetrical shape. Before, with her hair pulled back in a ponytail and straight bangs, the focus went predominantly to Rosie's nose.

We released the ponytail and used a flat-iron to create a subtle flip, added an off-center part and brushed her existing bangs to one side. Now attention flows to all her features equally and her face looks much more open and approachable. Statement earrings add presence to the whole look.

Getting Better Through the Years

Aging doesn't have to result in the stereotype of sagging, wrinkled skin and dowdy dress. We CAN get better as we get older. In the photos here you see a range of ages in several women who look better today than ever. Stay out of the sun and heed the skin care advice on page 147 to maintain your own healthy look for years to come. Update your hairstyle and wardrobe regularly with the strategies in this book—and you'll gain polish and self-confidence along the way.

A woman can continue to look good... or even better... as the years pass by.

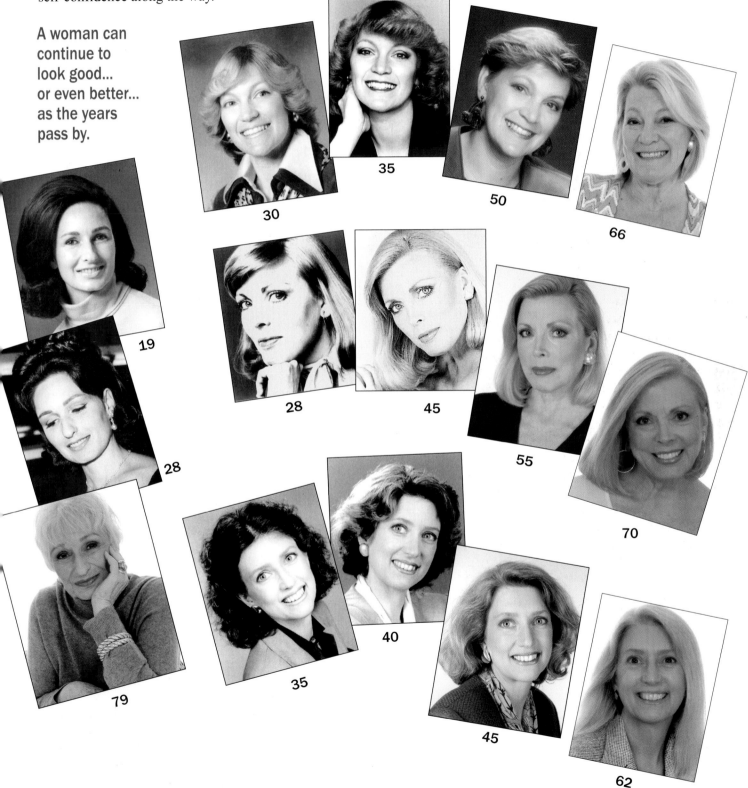

30

35

50

66

19

28

45

55

70

28

79

35

40

45

62

Chapter 15
Smart Shopping

Before You Shop, Become Fluent in Fashion

To win at wardrobe planning, learn to adapt what's in fashion this season to your personal appearance objectives. That may mean selecting a balance of classics, current trends, and perhaps an occasional fad.

The Fashion Curve

The direction in which fashion evolves can be plotted like this:

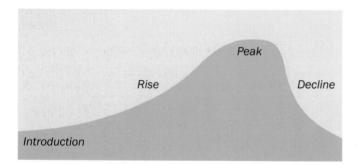

Introduction – A fashion trend is usually introduced in the runway shows of a high-fashion designer who creates one-of-a-kind styles. These are often too extreme for most consumers.

Rise – The designer trend is copied for mass production by high-end manufacturers. This style is featured in upscale retailers for elite clients at prices far lower than the designer's original.

Peak – The design is simplified and made with lesser fabrics and construction details to be widely distributed through mass retailers.

Decline – the look is so broadly distributed that everyone who wants it now owns it. It goes onto clearance racks and manufacturers stop producing it. The decline typically happens quickly compared with the rise.

Fashio-n trends probably evolve faster today due to instant communication.

Timing Your Purchases

A trendy item at its peak is one you may not be able to wear for long. One just beginning to rise may be a better buy. In other words, if you buy the style that everyone is wearing now, it could easily be out of fashion before you've gotten your money's worth of wear from it.

Sometimes we just don't get around to adding a new look as soon as we intended, and it's already past its peak. Or we spot a look we like, but realize it's just a short-lived fad. Add these items to your wardrobe only if you like them enough to enjoy their inherent value after their temporary spot in the limelight is past.

Fads and Classics

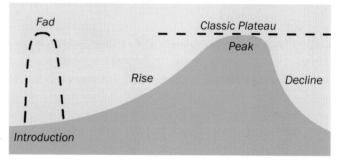

Both fads and classics have unique places along the fashion curve. Fads are short-lived styles that rise very quickly and decline with even greater speed. Fads are typically characterized by:

♦ Gimmicky details like nonfunctional pockets or buttons.

♦ Loud colors like chartreuse or iridescent orange.

♦ Extreme prints featuring bold colors and high-contrast combinations.

♦ Exaggerated details like very wide, oddly shaped collars or cuffs.

Classics are no-nonsense pieces that withstand influence from trends or fads. They are usually designed with clean, simple lines that allow you to adapt them to continuing style changes by varying the accessories or wearing the garments in different ways. Classics are reliable—never so "in" this season that they'll be "out" next year. They give you even more value for your money when they are beautifully constructed from high-quality fabrics in neutral colors.

Classic styles:

Sheath dresses
Cardigan jackets
Blazers
"Chanel" jackets
Slim skirts
Longer, soft skirts

Turtlenecks
Button-up shirts
Pullover sweaters
Trousers
Jeans

Classic details:

Set-in sleeves
Hems near the knee

Medium-width collars
  and lapels
Medium-width sleeves
Medium leg fullness

Do Your Fashion Homework

Early each season, do some snoop shopping to get ideas for what new color stories and design details are being featured. Whether you flip through magazines or catalogs, cruise the mall or surf the Internet, leave your charge cards in your wallet. This is an information gathering session. Make note of details like these:

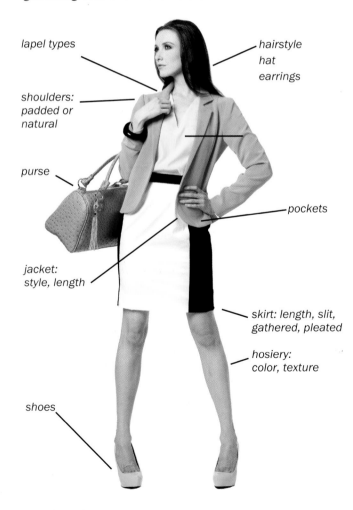

lapel types

hairstyle
hat
earrings

shoulders:
padded or
natural

purse

pockets

jacket:
style, length

skirt: length, slit,
gathered, pleated

hosiery:
color, texture

shoes

Get a seasonal overview from your armchair by skimming fashion magazines, catalogs and online style sites. Aa few good magazine choices are *Vogue, InStyle, Lucky, Harper's Bazaar,* and *W,* which also has an online "Mood Board" made up of their vast archive of photos. Visit the websites of your favorite retailers and sign up to receive their free catalogs (and you'll typically get coupons and invitations to special online sales too).

Remember that most of what magazines and style websites feature is the most extreme example of what's coming. By the time it reaches your local store it will be toned down to appeal to majority consumers.

Flip through the magazine, catalog or site pages, checking one detail at a time. Look at hemlines, for example. Then page through again noting shoulder lines and sleeves. Next time focus on colors … or whatever.

Pay special attention to accessories and how they are worn. And note hairstyles shown with newer fashions.

For each detail, consider how the trends you see relate to what you know about the colors, shapes and design details that flatter your body and face.

Create a valuable practice exercise by evaluating how well the clothes relate to the characteristics of the women modeling them. Surprisingly often the answer is "not very well."

Budget

Experts say most women wear 20 percent of their clothes 80 percent of the time. Our experience with clients indicates that 20 percent may be on the high side. But assuming it's accurate, learning to spend wisely and eliminate those mistakes—whether your budget is large or small—is equal to an 80% off sale on everything you select. Do yourself a big favor and use that savings to invest in higher quality items, even if they cost a little more.

Avoid impulse purchases by planning your wardrobe and budget in advance. Go through the last 12 months of your checkbook or charge statements and add up your wardrobe expenditures. The total may surprise you.

Then check your Needs List and estimate costs for each item. Make generous estimates rather than understating so you don't get trapped into buying poor-quality items just for their lower prices. All the better if you find a true bargain or two along the way and free up some funds for wardrobe extras.

Remember to budget for accessories too. Professionals advise clients to spend as much as a third of their budget for shoes, belts, scarves and jewelry to finish outfits with polish and pizzazz.

Plan your payment methods too. You can spread one shopping trip over several months' budgets by using a combination of cash or checks, charge cards and layaway.

Paying attention to seasonal sale dates, store discount coupons, and "friends and family" events can save you a third or more from regular retail prices of better in-season merchandise.

If your budget simply won't stretch to cover all your needs, decide which items can wait. Hope to find some things at end-of-season sales rather than settle for lesser-quality items that will look shoddy and wear out quickly. But be sure to shop those sales with the same discriminating eye you bring to full-price purchases.

156

A Fashion Dictionary

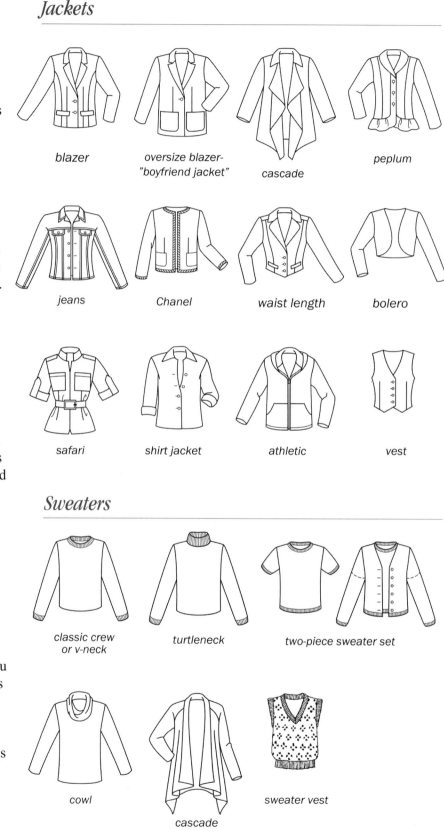

Jackets

blazer

oversize blazer-
"boyfriend jacket"

cascade

peplum

jeans

Chanel

waist length

bolero

safari

shirt jacket

athletic

vest

Sweaters

classic crew
or v-neck

turtleneck

two-piece sweater set

cowl

cascade

sweater vest

Blouses

classic shirt

camp shirt

classic blouse

shell

camisole

ruffled front with sleeves or sleeveless

wrapped

draped

baby doll (float)

T-shirts and Knit Tops

crew neck

V neck

tank

boat-neck

Henley

polo

cowl

deep draped

wrapped

Skirts

straight

contour waist

sarong

jeans skirt

A-line

wrap

design pleated

fully pleated

yoked

flared

gored, multi-panel

tiered

dirndl

Pants

pleated trouser

flat-front trouser

jeans

stirrup

legging

jeggings

pull-on, drawstring

capri

culotte

walking short

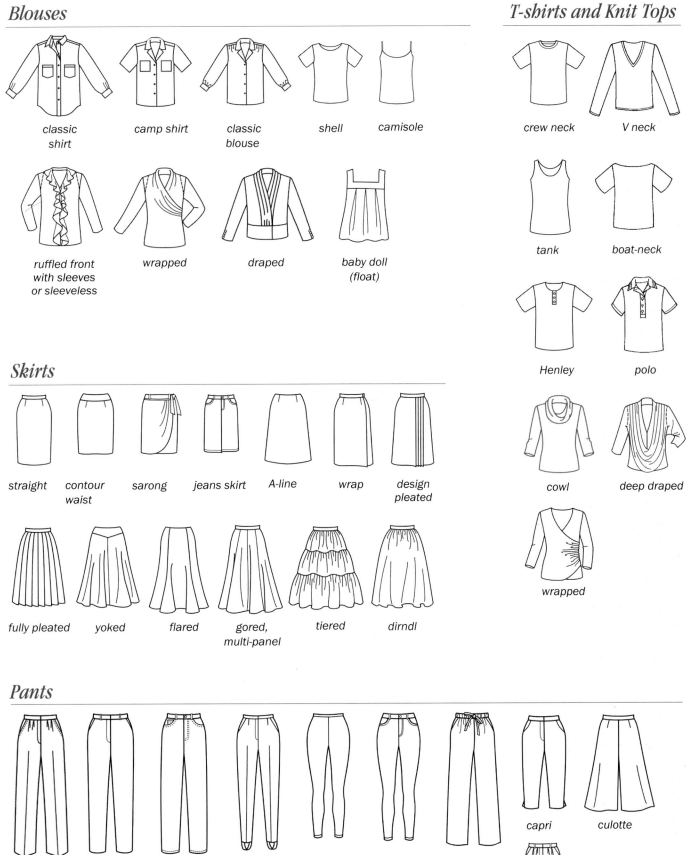

157

Dresses

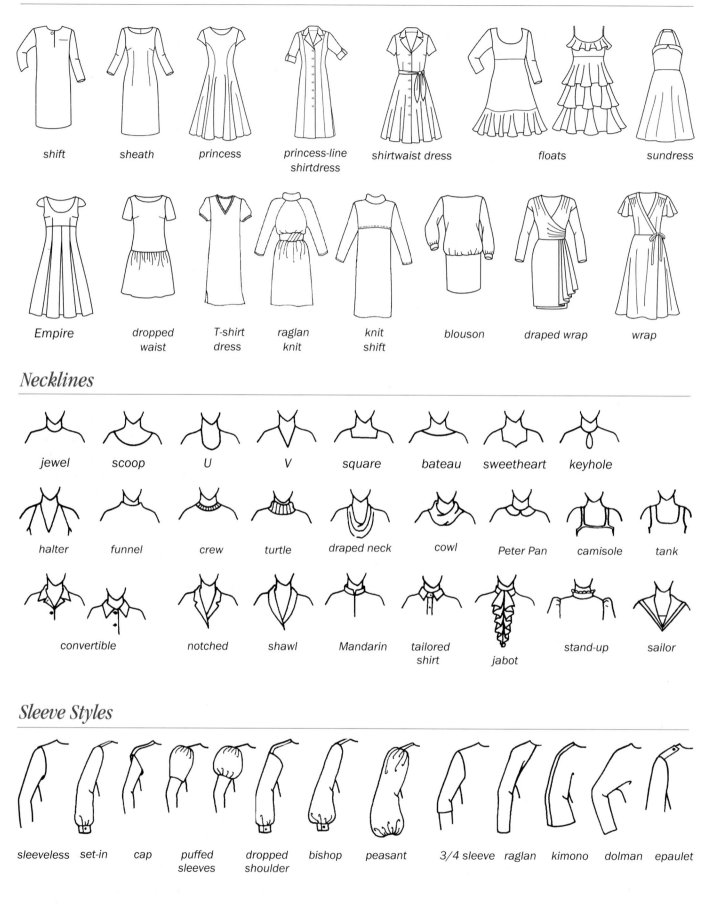

shift   sheath   princess   princess-line shirtdress   shirtwaist dress   floats   sundress

Empire   dropped waist   T-shirt dress   raglan knit   knit shift   blouson   draped wrap   wrap

Necklines

jewel   scoop   U   V   square   bateau   sweetheart   keyhole

halter   funnel   crew   turtle   draped neck   cowl   Peter Pan   camisole   tank

convertible   notched   shawl   Mandarin   tailored shirt   jabot   stand-up   sailor

Sleeve Styles

sleeveless   set-in   cap   puffed sleeves   dropped shoulder   bishop   peasant   3/4 sleeve   raglan   kimono   dolman   epaulet

158

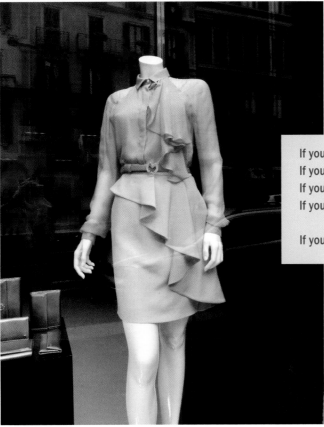

Window photo from Milan courtesy Lynn Weglarz

Shopping Smart

Snoop Shopping

Make time early in each season to explore the better stores for the trends you've spotted in magazines. This is an information gathering exercise, so leave your charge cards at home. Try on anything that catches your eye. Don't let price tags discourage you; you aren't buying today anyway.

Learning how more-expensive clothes fit and feel is a great education. You'll be a more discriminating consumer at more modest price levels. Or who knows —you may decide it's better to have fewer pieces but have them all be this fabulous.

Experiment with colors and styles you have learned should flatter you, but perhaps haven't tried yet. You may discover some great new looks by venturing just outside your normal comfort zone. Evaluate each look by standing as far as possible from a mirror to get the full effect. When an item seems close but not quite right, adapt it slightly by raising the hem a bit or tapering the skirt slightly before you finalize your opinion.

Make notes of what you liked, and what you didn't. Then go home and rest up for some serious shopping another day.

Retail Therapy

Women often jokingly refer to shopping as "retail therapy." In reality, shopping is the purposeful activity of obtaining needed additions to your wardrobe. Using shopping to meet emotional needs seldom leads to wise purchases.

If you want therapy...	work with a qualified counselor.
If you want to get out of the house...	take a healthy walk in the fresh air.
If you want stress relief...	listen to relaxing music.
If you want to socialize...	have coffee with a friend (even if it's while the kids are in Ronald's PlayPlace).
If you want to feel important...	volunteer in your community.

Only if you need an item for your wardrobe is shopping the answer.

Serious Shopping

Dress in good underwear, comfortable shoes (bring a pair of heels if you'll be trying on dressier clothes), and easy-off clothing. We recommend shopping solo, unless you're working with a professional wardrobe consultant. Your friends, bless their hearts, will lie to you. Who wants to tell her best pal that yes indeed, that does make your butt look fat? And friends sometimes get their shopping fix from your purchases, making them less likely to provide the voice of reason.

Be sure to take:

♦ Your color fan
♦ Your inventory of current clothes
♦ Your Needs List
♦ Items you need to match

"Top Down" Shopping

Plan to buy the very best quality you can afford. Remember, you're worth full price. Many women find this philosophy hard to embrace at first. We can become so caught up in the momentary rush of so-called "bargain" purchases that we never experience the lasting joy of owning truly wonderful things. Those wonderful things are often the real bargains, as we continue to use and delight in them for years.

Even if your budget is tight, start this shopping expedition at a store a notch or two above your normal price point. Remember the 80/20 concept. If you shop right you'll need fewer pieces, so you really can pay more without spending more. You'll learn important lessons about fit and quality in the process. And the higher prices help you avoid buying more items than you really need.

Bargains are great, but only if the item is great for you first. **You are worth full price!** If, as you shop down the price scale, you find a truly equal substitute for one of your more expensive purchases, feel free to make the switch knowing that you've found a great value, not just a low price.

Wherever you shop, resolve never to buy an item if:

- It's at the end of its fashion curve.
- It won't work at least three ways in your wardrobe.
- Its only appeal is the sale price.

Here are some shopping venues to consider, listed in roughly descending order by price point:

- **Direct sale trunk shows** offer designer clothing in a private environment hosted by a trained consultant. The collections are typically well-coordinated to make wardrobe building easier. In an individual appointment, you see and touch actual samples, then order your size direct from the company. Although you may not be able to try on your chosen style in your size, consultants are trained to help you approximate the look and calculate the size to order. And exchanges are usually available at no cost. These companies typically offer extensive size ranges, perhaps 0-18, and sell tops and bottoms separately, so they can accommodate a wide range of figures. Trunk shows range from mid-price to upper levels.

- **Specialty clothing stores**—from Neiman Marcus, Saks and Nordstrom on the high end to Ann Taylor, Talbots and Chico's in the more moderate price range—also offer good color coordination and selection in a pleasant shopping environment. Sales personnel are usually knowledgeable about the merchandise selection and quick to suggest coordinated pieces. These retailers often offer customer loyalty programs that reward regular shoppers with discounts and special events, so it pays to identify a favorite or two and shop with them consistently. This category also includes stores that cater to special sizes like plus, petite, and tall.

- **Department stores** offer large selection and the ability to ship merchandise from other locations if your favorite item is sold out in your size. Because they carry similar merchandise in misses, plus and petite sizing, department stores are a big help to women who need different sizing for different parts of their bodies. They also feature temporary markdowns on in-season merchandise and special coupon promotions to reduce your cost further. Apply for a store charge card to get advance notice. Then go to the store the night before the event; often the discounts are loaded into the computerized registers before the home office closes at 5 p.m., so you can buy at sale prices and beat the crowds. If not, you'll still be able to browse, try on and make choices in relative calm, and have your selections held for pickup the next day.

On the minus side, department stores are often short-staffed and often move salespeople from department to department to fill staffing gaps.

- **Off-price retailers** like Marshalls/T.J. Maxx, Stein Mart, and outlet malls sometimes have nice merchandise at considerable savings.

It works this way: A manufacturer cuts a quantity of a particular design. Their retailer clients buy most of that quantity. The leftover pieces are sold to an off-price chain, which gets a sizable discount in exchange for taking whatever assortment the manufacturer has on hand. Or the items go directly to the manufacturer's own outlet operation.

Off-price and outlet stores operate in no-frills locations with minimal staffing to keep overhead—and therefore pricing—low. The selection typically includes broken sizing or only some pieces from coordinated groupings. New merchandise arrives frequently. It can take real effort to unearth bargains, but some women are willing to invest the time or simply enjoy the thrill of the hunt.

A few cautions about off-price shopping:

- Check store policies about checks and charges, exchanges and returns. They are often more limiting than conventional retailers' policies.

- Check quality carefully since manufacturers dispose of their irregulars and seconds through these same channels.

- Be discriminating. These stores get merchandise from poor-quality manufacturers as well as fine brand names. Don't get carried away by low prices. It's only a bargain if it's the perfect item for you and your wardrobe.

- Brand-name outlet stores often carry merchandise made specifically for this lower-price environment. They have a look similar to the company's full-price line, but with compromises in fabric quality, style details, or quality construction.

♦ **Nicer resale shops** can be a source of some almost unbelievable bargains. Seek out ones that carry superior quality, little-worn garments. Some of the best are sponsored by women's civic and charitable organizations and located in affluent areas. Obviously the selection and sizes are totally hit and miss. And returns are not usually an option.

♦ **Discount retailers** (Walmart, H&M, Forever 21) offer ultra-low pricing that isn't usually a true bargain. The quality of the fabrics and the construction are not usually up to standard. And the conditions in third-world factories are questionable at best. When a price tag seems too good to be true, something is usually amiss. We recommend spending a bit more to buy quality garments you can wear with pride, even if it means buying fewer items each season.

Three other options defy classification in our price point strata, but merit special mention.

♦ **Online and catalog shopping.** Ease and selection are the upsides here. Inability to try on sizes, compare colors or inspect quality are obvious minuses. In general, we consider these to be good resources for pre-shopping, but prefer to spend our dollars supporting local retailers whenever possible.

♦ **Specialty boutiques** offer relatively limited selection, but often more distinctive styles than you'll see in conventional stores. The merchandise usually reflects the particular style viewpoint of the owner, so when you find a retailer whose taste mirrors your own the result can be very exciting. Price and quality levels in boutiques vary widely.

♦ **Custom sewing**—either for yourself or by a professional dressmaker—is an effective way to get exactly the style, color, fit, and fabric you want for your wardrobe additions. You can locate a highly qualified sewing professional through the Association of Sewing and Design Professionals at www.sewingprofessionals.org.

Cost-per-Wear Formula

To decide if a particular item is a good investment, consider its cost per wearing instead of the number on the price tag. Add the initial cost plus anticipated maintenance (alterations, routine dry cleaning, etc.). Calculate how many times you expect to wear it. Divide the first number by the second to determine cost per wearing.

COST-PER-WEAR EXAMPLE 1:
Winter coat costs $300 and will require annual dry cleaning for $25. If you wear the coat 5 times a week for 26 cold weeks each year and keep it for 3 years, that's 390 wearings. Price plus cleaning equals $375.

$375 divided by 390 = $0.96 per wearing

Well worth the big initial spend.

COST-PER-WEAR EXAMPLE 2:
Sequined cocktail dress marked down from $295 to $99.99. You can wear it to two parties this year and two occasions next year before everyone in your social circle has seen it.

$100 divided by 4 = $25 per wearing

A relatively pricey choice. A mix and match group of dressy separates might be a wiser use of your money. See page 106.

Sanity-Saving Shopping Strategies

♦ Shop early in the season while selection is at its best. Seasons in retail are well ahead of the calendar and the thermometer, as any woman who has tried to buy a swimsuit in July has quickly discovered. Spring merchandise arrives in stores as the ball is dropping in Times Square; fall clothes are on the racks before the Fourth of July fireworks have fallen back to earth. Watch for pre-season pricing specials if you must, but get your must-have wardrobe additions while the getting is good.

♦ If you love shopping the clearance rack, use it as a chance to add fun extras to your wardrobe. Finding basics there is unlikely, especially in best-selling middle sizes.

♦ Shop when stores are least crowded—weekday mornings, dinnertime, and in bad weather. If you must shop on weekends, get in and out early.

♦ Consistently shop a few favorite stores so you can develop relationships with salespeople. They'll call you with word of new arrivals and impending markdowns.

♦ Never shop at the last minute for a big event. You'll invariably be forced into an emergency purchase that isn't likely to work well in the long run.

♦ Always shop with your color fan. Don't even try on anything that isn't in your best range. You'll be amazed how much you'll speed up your shopping.

♦ Create a swatch file of your current clothes to take along when you shop. Mobile phone and tablet apps like Stylebook and others guarantee that you won't leave home without your virtual wardrobe.

♦ Experiment. Try on things you're not sure about, if they meet your color and silhouette criteria. We love it when shopping clients tell us, "I never would have tried that on my own … and I love it!"

♦ Get over the size obsession. Take at least two sizes of an item to the fitting room, and try on both without checking the tags. Buy the one that fits better. Nobody will ever see the number, but everybody will see how it looks on your body.

♦ If the store has more than one in your size, try them all. Clothes are cut by machines, but sewn by humans. Even a tiny difference in seam depth can noticeably change the fit.

♦ Expect alterations. Standard clothing sizes can't provide instant fit for the huge variety of female bodies. Work with an alterations specialist to customize hems, sleeve length, and other fit details. You'll look better proportioned and your clothes will look more expensive too.

♦ Find underwear, pantyhose and other basics that you like, and then wait for sales to stock up big. You can even order by phone or online.

♦ If you really hate shopping, have it done for you. Better stores have shopping services at no charge. Call in your list and let them do the footwork for you. All you do is try on and make final selections. Be aware that store personal shoppers are commissioned salespeople and may not be trained in "points of connection" concepts.

♦ Freelance personal shoppers provide a similar service for an hourly fee and aren't limited to any one store's merchandise. Interview a personal shopper thoroughly to be sure he or she is not just trend-aware, but also thoroughly knowledgeable in color, line, design, scale, and so on.

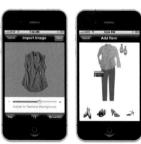 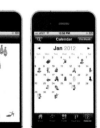

Photos compliments of Stylebook.

Quality Checkpoints

Always buy the very best quality you can afford. It is a false economy to do anything else, since cheaper items wear out quickly, and the replacement next year will almost always cost more. The cheap item will never look as good or feel as luxurious on your body as the finer garment. Here are some guidelines to help you recognize quality in garment construction regardless of the price.

Quality Check Chart—Look for These Details:

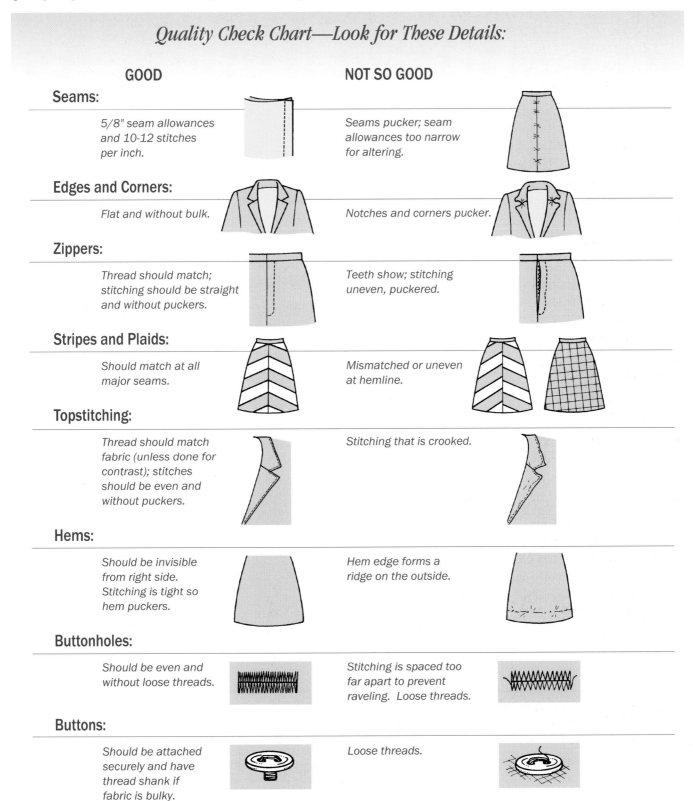

	GOOD	NOT SO GOOD
Seams:	5/8" seam allowances and 10-12 stitches per inch.	Seams pucker; seam allowances too narrow for altering.
Edges and Corners:	Flat and without bulk.	Notches and corners pucker.
Zippers:	Thread should match; stitching should be straight and without puckers.	Teeth show; stitching uneven, puckered.
Stripes and Plaids:	Should match at all major seams.	Mismatched or uneven at hemline.
Topstitching:	Thread should match fabric (unless done for contrast); stitches should be even and without puckers.	Stitching that is crooked.
Hems:	Should be invisible from right side. Stitching is tight so hem puckers.	Hem edge forms a ridge on the outside.
Buttonholes:	Should be even and without loose threads.	Stitching is spaced too far apart to prevent raveling. Loose threads.
Buttons:	Should be attached securely and have thread shank if fabric is bulky.	Loose threads.

What Is Good Fit?

Excellent fit means more than just "I can zip it." It means the garment flows gracefully over your body without pulling or binding, sagging or bagging. It means that garment details like darts, shaping seams, and hems fall at the ideal level.

Bad fit gets your attention as soon as you slip a garment on. You find yourself tugging, wiggling, and twisting in a fruitless attempt to get comfortable in it. Uncorrected, bad fit ultimately gets everyone else's attention too.

Many women confuse sizing with fitting. *Sizing* means finding the standard garment that gives you enough fabric around your critical fit dimension—the largest body area the garment will cover. *Fit* means customizing that standard garment for all the details of your shape. Buying pants that fit your hips would be a sizing decision. Having them shortened for your height and taken in for your proportionally smaller waist would be a fitting exercise.

You can simplify the fitting process by shopping in the departments that provide sizing closest to your needs:

♦ Misses sizes fit women over about 5'5".

♦ Petite sizes fit women 5'4" and under. But a taller woman with proportionally shorter legs might buy petite pants and skirts to wear with her misses jackets. Or a short-waisted woman might need petite jackets to wear with her misses bottoms. A petite size is typically one notch smaller than the same number size in misses, so a misses 8 is generally equal to a petite 10.

♦ Women's sizes are shaped for a somewhat thicker body. A women's size 12 is roughly equal to a misses 18, but shaped more generously. A woman with a thicker torso might choose bottoms in misses' sizes and tops in the women's department.

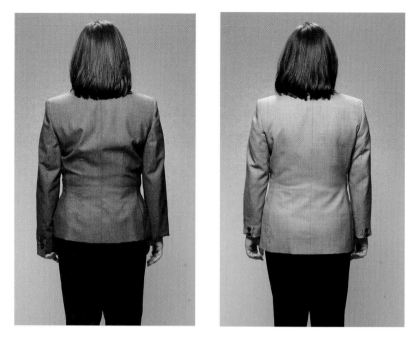

This woman, 5'6" tall, struggled to find jackets that didn't bunch up across the back. She was surprised to discover that, because her body is short from shoulder to waist, she got a much-improved fit in a jacket from the Petite department. By choosing separates, she can still purchase coordinating skirts and pants in Misses sizing.

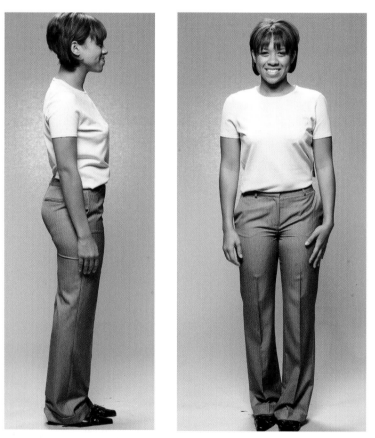

These examples show many ways to identify a too-tight fit in pants—cupping tightly under the derriere and tummy, showing panty lines, pulling the creases smooth over the thighs, angled pockets bowing open, horizontal and diagonal wrinkles pulling across the front. A larger size, with gently skimming fit, would actually make her body look trimmer.

Good Fit Checkpoint

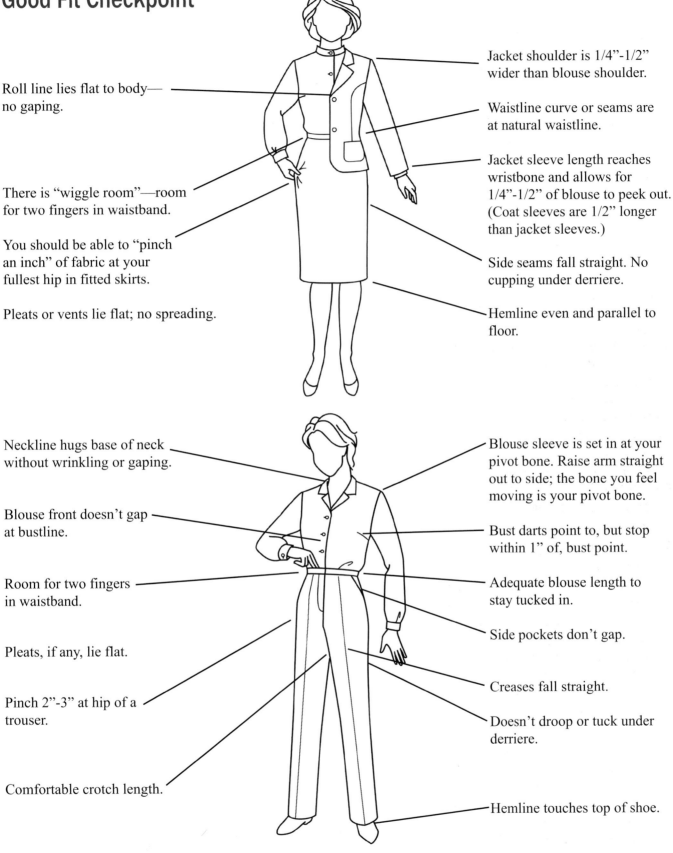

Roll line lies flat to body—no gaping.

There is "wiggle room"—room for two fingers in waistband.

You should be able to "pinch an inch" of fabric at your fullest hip in fitted skirts.

Pleats or vents lie flat; no spreading.

Jacket shoulder is 1/4"-1/2" wider than blouse shoulder.

Waistline curve or seams are at natural waistline.

Jacket sleeve length reaches wristbone and allows for 1/4"-1/2" of blouse to peek out. (Coat sleeves are 1/2" longer than jacket sleeves.)

Side seams fall straight. No cupping under derriere.

Hemline even and parallel to floor.

Neckline hugs base of neck without wrinkling or gaping.

Blouse front doesn't gap at bustline.

Room for two fingers in waistband.

Pleats, if any, lie flat.

Pinch 2"-3" at hip of a trouser.

Comfortable crotch length.

Blouse sleeve is set in at your pivot bone. Raise arm straight out to side; the bone you feel moving is your pivot bone.

Bust darts point to, but stop within 1" of, bust point.

Adequate blouse length to stay tucked in.

Side pockets don't gap.

Creases fall straight.

Doesn't droop or tuck under derriere.

Hemline touches top of shoe.

Test the fit both standing and seated. Can you move freely in the garment?
Bend arms and lift them over your head.

Fabric Fundamentals

A few basic fabric facts can help you make sure that the great-looking garment in the store is an equally great performer in your wardrobe.

Fiber Facts

1. Fiber absorbency is a clue to comfort and durability.

   - More-absorbent fibers are more comfortable to wear because they absorb body moisture and humidity. They are less prone to static electricity and will clean more easily.

   - Less-absorbent fibers are less affected by body heat and moisture. They wrinkle less and hold their shape better. But they are less comfortable, more static prone, and they pill more easily.

   Synthetic fibers like polyester, nylon, acetate and acrylic are less absorbent. Natural fibers like wool, linen, cotton and silk are more absorbent. Rayon, though technically a synthetic, is made from plant cellulose so it behaves more like a natural fiber.

2. The length of a fiber also affects appearance and performance of fabrics.

   - Long fibers are smooth and lustrous, wrinkle resistant, and pill resistant. Synthetics and natural silk are long fibers. The finest cotton and wool fibers are also relatively long.

   - Short fibers are soft and fuzzy, tend to pill, and wrinkle more easily. Most natural fibers are short, and some synthetics are cut into short lengths for a more natural appearance.

3. Manufacturers often blend fibers to decrease costs, increase prestige, increase washability, minimize wrinkling, or add comfort and strength. It generally takes 35 percent of a fiber in a blend to make a significant difference, and 50 percent to get the most out of that fiber's good qualities. (An exception is spandex fiber such as Lycra, since 5% will add significant stretch.)

   - A shirt of 65 percent cotton, 35 percent polyester will wrinkle less and wear better than an all-cotton shirt.

   - A blend of opposite proportions (65 percent polyester, 35 percent cotton) will wrinkle even less and wear even longer, but will also be less comfortable to wear.

These fibers in a fabric...	contribute...
Cotton or linen	Absorbency and comfort, minimum static buildup, better dyeability
Wool	Bulk and warmth, absorbency, shape retention, wrinkle recovery
Silk	Luster, luxury, comfort
Mohair	Strength, luster, loopy texture
Cashmere/camel hair	Warmth, luxury, drapability, softness
Angora	Softness, fuzziness
Acrylic	Softness, wool-like qualities
Rayon and bamboo	Absorbency, low static buildup, luster
Nylon	Strength, abrasion resistance, wrinkle resistance, lower cost
Acetate	Drapability, luster and shine, lower cost
Polyester	Wash-and-wear qualities, wrinkle resistance, shape retention, lower cost
Spandex	Elasticity and comfort

If you are unsure about care instructions, care as you would for the most sensitive fiber in the blend.

4. Fabric weave also affects durability and appearance.

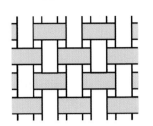

- **Plain weave** – Each crosswise thead runs over one lengthwise thread, then under the next, producing a strong, firm fabric of any weight. Broadcloth, challis, chiffon, and flannel are examples of this most common weave.

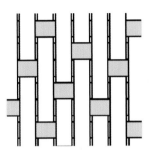

- **Satin weave** – Lengthwise threads "float" over several crosswise threads before going under one, to produce very lustrous fabric. These float yarns can snag easily. Charmeuse and satin are examples of this more fragile weave.

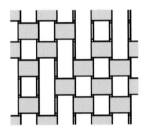

- **Jacquard/dobby weaves** – Figurative designs are produced by patterns of float threads, making some of the areas of the fabric shinier. These are expensive to produce and can be fragile. Brocade is an example.

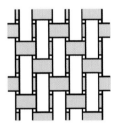

- **Twill weave** – A fine diagonal rib is formed in this strong, wrinkle-resistant weave. Examples are denim and gabardine.

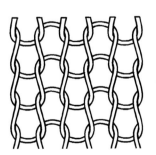

- **Knits** – The yarn is formed into a series of interlocking loops. Knits are durable, but subject to snags. They are comfortable because of their stretchability.

  Single knits curl along the cut edge. Double knits are more weighty and do not curl or run.

How Can I Tell if This Fabric Will Work for Me?

- Test wrinkle resistance and recovery by crushing a corner of fabric in your hand and releasing it. Do the wrinkles stay or fall out quickly? The higher the natural fiber content, the more it will wrinkle. Woven fabrics wrinkle more than knits. Ask yourself if some wrinkles are a fair trade for the look the fabric gives to the garment.

- Check wearing qualities and shape retention. Stretch the fabric between thumbs and forefingers and hold for five seconds. If the yarns shift apart, strain on seams could be a problem when you wear the garment. If the fabric doesn't spring back, the garment may stretch out of shape in wearing. Generally woven fabrics hold their shape better than knits, and synthetics better than natural fibers.

- Test the fabric for pilling. In an inconspicuous area of the garment, gently rub two layers of fabric right sides together. If this produces slight balls of fibers (called pills), the same thing will happen in abrasion areas when you wear the garment.

- Check the fiber content for a comfort guide. In general, fabrics high in natural fibers are more comfortable. Synthetics often feel clammy because they don't breathe or absorb as well.

- Check grain line. Lengthwise and crosswise threads should be at right angles to one another and lengthwise threads should run straight up and down the garment. Otherwise the garment will not hang evenly on your body.

Invest in the best quality you can afford for your wardrobe basics. These coordinates need to be durable and make you look like a million.

Fabrics for Basic Skirts/Jackets/Pants

Fabric	Advantages	Disadvantages
Wool Gabardine	Wears extremely well. Comfortable because wool breathes and insulates. Lightweight gabs are seasonless, hold shape well, wrinkles hang out.	Expensive. Easily over-pressed. *Dry clean only.*
Wool Crepe	Drapes beautifully. Season-spanning comfort. Wrinkles hang out.	Expensive. Can snag. *Dry clean.*
Polyester Gabardine	Wrinkle-resistant, durable. Year-round wear except in hottest/coldest climates. Stays crisp, fresh. *Washable.*	Not quite as rich-looking as wool. Can snag or pill. Less comfortable than wool.
Linen and Silk Suitings	Generally wear well. Never pill. Absorbent and very comfortable. Dark colors are seasonless.	Lose body after repeated cleaning; use spray sizing to restore body. Dark colors show wear more quickly. *Dry Clean.*
Linen-like	Choose heavier weights for better wear. Blends of rayon, polyester, cotton, and/or linen are less costly and more wrinkle-resistant than pure linen. *Washable.*	May pill. Loses body after washing or dry cleaning. Not as durable or rich-looking as pure linen. *Line dry because dryer can cause pilling.*

Fabrics for Soft Skirts & Blouses

Fabric	Advantages	Disadvantages
Polyester Crepe de Chine	Drapes beautifully for fullness without bulk. Resists wrinkles. Very durable. *Machine wash.*	Nonabsorbent, can feel clammy. Subject to oily stains. Remove from dryer promptly to prevent heat-set wrinkles.
Silk Crepe de Chine	Superb drape and feel. Comfortable in all climates. Prints and dyes beautifully.	Expensive. Subject to perspiration stains and damage. Wrinkles. *Hand wash or dryclean.*
Silk Broadcloth	Sportier, crisper, and stronger than crepe de chine. Less expensive.	Susceptible to wrinkles and perspiration damage. *Hand wash or dry clean.*
Silk Charmeuse	Shiny surface and soft drape. Dressy.	Can snag. *Dry clean.*
Cotton or Blended Broadcloth	More casual. Inexpensive. More comfortable than polyester. Wrinkles less than silk. *Washable.*	Higher cotton content, wrinkles more; higher polyester content, less comfortable.
Wool or Blend Challis	Lightweight and drapable. Usually a soft, warm, brushed surface. *Most blends wash well.*	Wool is more expensive, but durable. Polyester has tendency to pill. *Dry clean pure wool.*
Rayon Challis	Beautiful drape. Comfortable for year-round wear. *Usually washable.*	Retains new look longer if *dry cleaned.*

Additional Fabrics for Added Variety

Fabric	Advantages	Disadvantages
Wool and Blended Flannel	Those with tight weave or hard finish wear best. Good winter basic in weights for all climates. *Blends* usually less expensive and *washable.*	Generally for winter only. Can be expensive. Less durable and more wrinkly than gabardine. Blends can pill or be scratchy. *Dry clean 100 percent wool.*
Wool Knit	Comfortable. Warm in winter. Lightweights drape beautifully. Heavier weights tailor well. *Sweaters may be hand washed.*	Expensive. Can snag. May stretch out of shape in wear, but can be pressed back. *Dry clean.*
Polyester Knit	Resists wrinkles; travels well. Holds its shape. Inexpensive. *Machine washable.*	Fiber doesn't breathe, so warm in summer; cold in winter. Subject to snags and oily stains.
Corduroy, Velvet, and Velveteen	Very rich texture and color. *Some are washable.*	Not very durable; show wear and press marks easily. Can stretch out of shape, but will recover in washing or *dry cleaning.*

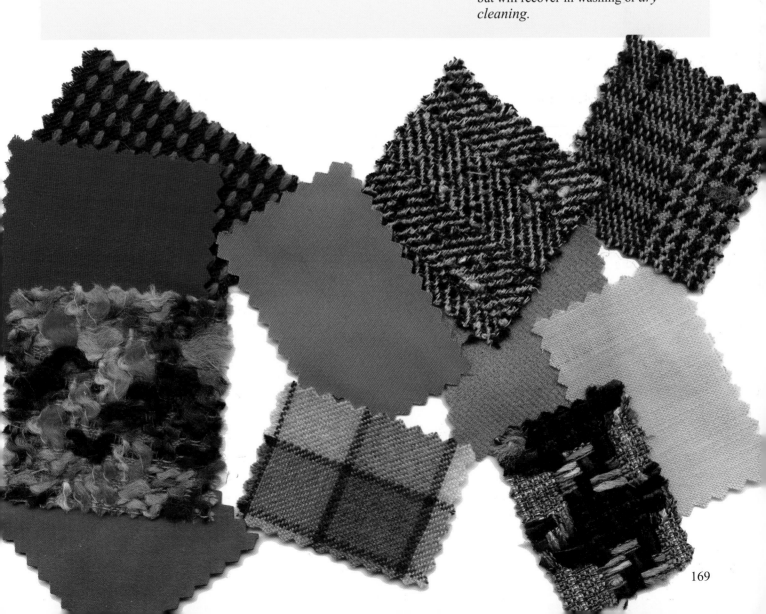

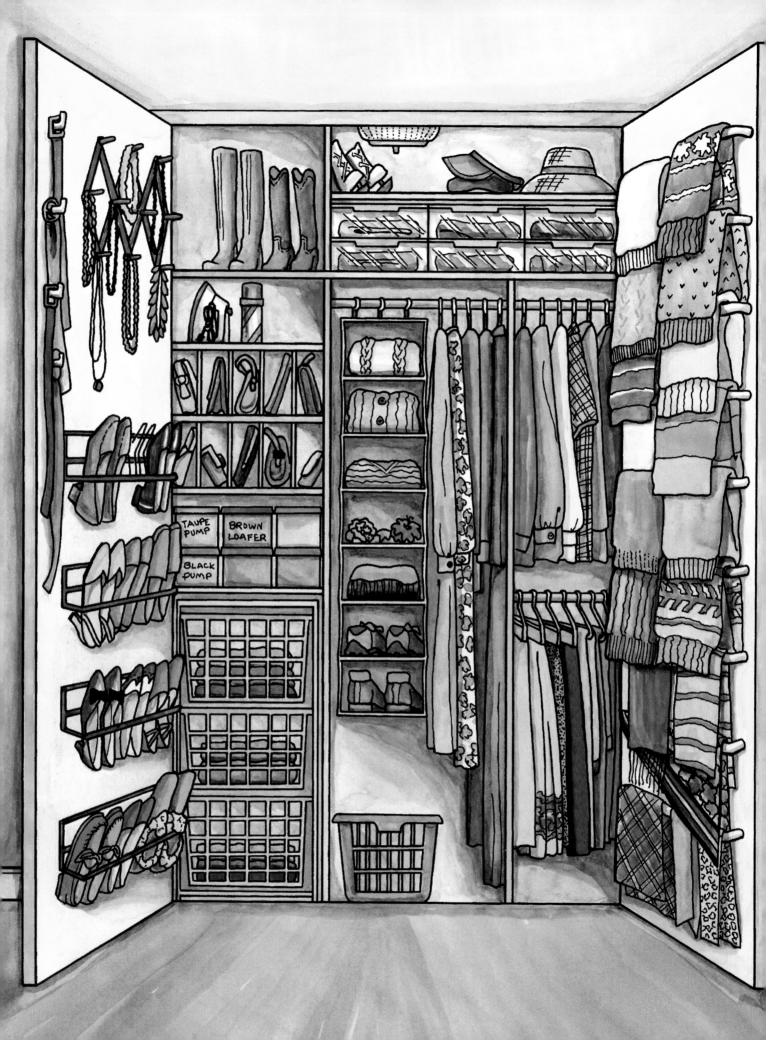

Chapter 16
Closet Control

Get Organized

It's much easier to get dressed in the morning if your closet is organized and everything is visible. And, you'll start every day with the calm, Zen-like feeling of being surrounded by lovely color harmony. It's a no-cost luxury every woman deserves.

♦ Hang everything. You are far less likely to remember and use items that are hidden away in drawers.

♦ Hang each garment individually. The exceptions would be suits or two-piece dresses that you would never wear except as a matched set.

♦ Create two hanging levels so you can see your tops in relation to your bottoms. You'll be amazed how many more combinations you'll see immediately. And how much more space you'll have in your closet. Buy a hanging system or make your own with screw eyes, S-hooks, chain and dowels.

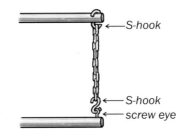

← S-hook

← S-hook
← screw eye

♦ Use the inside of doors for extra hanging space. Add a towel bar for scarves, a shoe rack, or a row of cup hooks for belts or jewelry.

♦ Make your closet light and bright with a fresh coat of light-colored paint. Mix a bit of your bedroom wall color into plain white paint for a custom coordinated look.

♦ Make the most of your closet lighting. Remove a frosted cover to get the full wattage of the bulbs.

♦ Or wire a multi-bulb fixture—the kind you find over a bathroom mirror—into the single ceiling outlet. Check local electrical codes, though, to be sure your new lighting will meet safety standards.

♦ To avoid faded garments, always turn off lights when you close the closet.

♦ No wiring? Install a battery-operated light instead.

♦ Organize all your clothes by categories. See page 89 for more detail.

♦ In a two-tier arrangement, hang skirts and pants on the top rod. Although it may seem backwards, this arrangement lets more overhead light filter through to the blouses and jackets hanging below.

♦ Organize each category in color order—neutrals first, light to dark, then all the colors in rainbow sequence—red, orange, yellow, green, blue, purple.

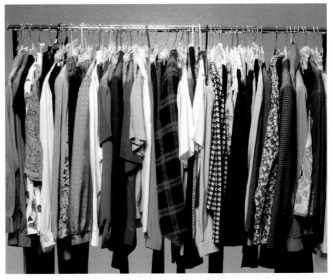

Sue's BEFORE closet contents are excessive, uncoordinated, and disorganized. No wonder she feels she has nothing to wear.

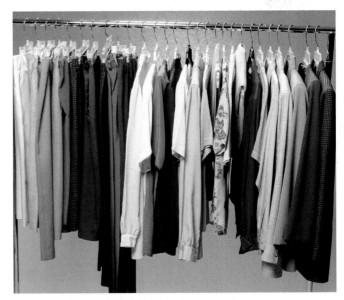

After some serious editing (see pages 86-87 for guidelines) and re-organizing, Sue's AFTER closet will be soothing to look at and much easier to use. It's hard to believe, but everything here was also in the BEFORE closet. In a closet, truly "less is more."

Safe Storage Strategies

Here are some tips to minimize closet wear and tear on your wardrobe.

♦ Don't crowd your closet. Let clothes hang freely to prevent wrinkling.

♦ Take all your wire hangers back to the dry cleaner for recycling and replace them with one of these:

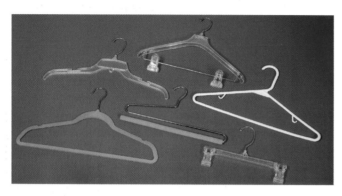

♦ Loops of ribbon sewn into the waistline of some dresses are intended to slip over the hanger hook to support the weight of the garment and prevent shoulder distortion or lengthwise stretching. You can add them to other garments yourself.

♦ Keep fragile items like lace, beaded items, velvet, and suede in cloth bags for protection. Avoid plastic bags, which don't let the fabric breathe.

♦ You can store sweaters right on hangers (see page 89). Avoid hanging fuzzy fabrics like mohair or fur next to ones that attract lint.

♦ Clip-style skirt hangers can leave indentations on fine fabrics. Protect your garment by tucking a scrap of medium-weight fabric between the waistband and the clips.

Storage Solutions

Here are some specific ideas for hard-to-manage items:

Hang belts from:

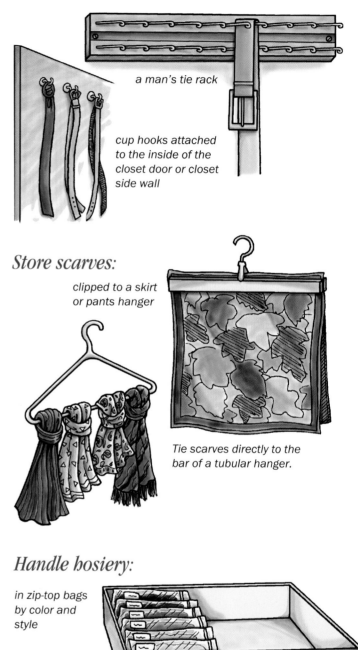

a man's tie rack

cup hooks attached to the inside of the closet door or closet side wall

Store scarves:

clipped to a skirt or pants hanger

Tie scarves directly to the bar of a tubular hanger.

Handle hosiery:

in zip-top bags by color and style

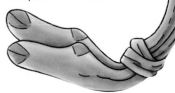

Knot pairs with runs to identify them for wear with pants or boots.

For jewelry:

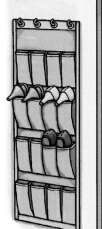

mug rack

cup hooks

cutlery tray

styrofoam egg carton

plastic compartmented box

mesh pencil cup

ribbon strip for pins or silk flowers

hanging organizer

Store shoes on:

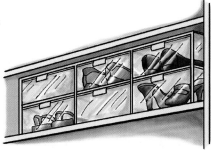

shelves in see-through plastic boxes or shoe boxes with photos or written labels on the outside

freestanding or door-mounted racks

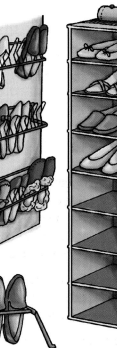

Boots can hang from clips of a pant hanger to prevent folds at the ankle, or use boot inserts. Make sure the clips on the hanger do not damage the leather—a piece of spongy material tucked over the edge of the boots can help.

Handbags can go:

- between vertical dividers on a shelf.
- in freestanding wire baskets.
- in a hanging purse/shoe caddy.
- hung by their handles from ceiling-mounted hooks (think of a kitchen pot rack).

Out-of-Season Storage

- Store clothes in cool, dry areas to prevent mildew and out of direct sunlight to guard against fading.

- Create storage space by adding an extra-high rod in a tall closet or a back rod in a deep closet.

- Garment racks and storage boxes can expand available space.

- Furs need professional reconditioning and cold storage off-season to prevent drying and cracking.

- Mothproofing is a MUST when temperatures exceed 50 degrees. Scatter moth balls liberally through stored items. Use layers of tissue paper to protect fabric from direct contact with mothballs. Keep the storage area sealed tight to hold in the vapors. NOTE: Don't use moth balls with leathers or furs.

- If you can't stand the mothball smell, substitute cedar blocks or make one of these herbal blends instead. You'll find the ingredients at health food or craft stores. These mixes don't kill moth larvae but they will repel egg-laying moths. In your blender, make a powder from equal parts of:

MIX 1	MIX 2	MIX 3
Sassafras	Thyme	Cloves
Lavender	Lavender	Caraway seeds
Dried rue	Woodruff	Nutmeg
Rosemary	Mace	Cinnamon

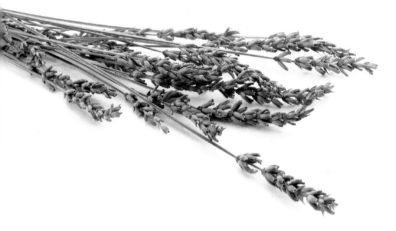

Clothing Care

Quality clothes are worth protecting for longer life and better looks.

- Air out clothes. Hang them outside the closet overnight so wrinkles fall out and odors dissipate. Dropping them in a pile results in more frequent cleaning, which causes unnecessary wear and expense.

- Brush clothes to get rid of fiber-breaking dust… then dry clean only occasionally.

- Let your clothes rest between wearings to regain their shape.

- Mend small tears immediately before they develop into bigger ones.

- Remove pills with a "de-fuzzer" or whisk Dr. Scholl's callous remover gently over the surface of the fabric.

- Use a snag repair tool (found in fabric stores) to pull a snagged thread through to the wrong side of a garment.

- To recover stretched-out sweater cuffs, dampen them by rolling in a wet washcloth, then tumble in the dryer for a few minutes.

- Let your deodorant, perfume, and lotions dry completely before you dress. These products contain chemicals that can damage fibers.

- Stop runs in panty hose with clear nail polish or Fray Check clear ravel preventer (found in fabric stores). Paint the toe seam with Fray Check before wearing to prolong their life.

- Use an emery file to smooth rough edges on the back of jewelry to prevent snagging clothes.

Removing Stains

- Most spots can be removed completely with immediate action. The longer a spot sits, the harder it is to remove.

- Never press over a spot; heat is likely to set the stain permanently.

- Keep a spot remover on hand for quick saves on dry cleaning. Test in an inconspicuous area of the garment first.

- Waiters and flight attendants swear by club soda to prevent stains from setting.

- To remove a stain, put a clean towel under the fabric, with the stain toward the cloth. Use soft absorbent fabric to dab stain remover or water through the stain until it is gone.

Perspiration – On washables, pretreat by flushing with an ammonia/water solution. Rinse well.

Ink – Water-soluble hair spray dissolves ink on washables. Use rubbing alcohol on dry clean fabrics.

Oils – On silks, pretreat and wash with Easy Wash. On polyesters, pretreat with Spray 'N' Wash and launder.

Wash or Dry Clean?

Read and follow the manufacturer's care label. Often a garment in a fabric you'd expect to be washable requires dry cleaning because of the interfacings or linings used inside.

Among washables, the more delicate the fabric the more likely it should be hand washed and air dried rather than laundered and dried by machine.

Hand Washing Silk

1. To lukewarm water (100 degrees), add a mild shampoo. Silk is protein, like hair. Or use a cold-water detergent like Wool Tone by Van Wyck.

2. Swish the garment through the solution for 1-2 minutes. Don't rub, twist or wring.

3. Rinse thoroughly in cold water (50 degrees) to remove soap and minimize wrinkling.

4. Lay wet garment on a towel and roll up to blot excess water.

5. Use a dry iron at low temperature to gently iron the garment dry.

Hand Washing Sweaters

1. To cool water, add a cold-water detergent like Wool Tone.

2. Very gently squeeze soapy water through the sweater for just 1-2 minutes, no more. Rinse twice in cold water.

3. Pat out water, and then roll in a towel to blot excess moisture.

4. Dry sweater flat, blocking to original size if needed.

Machine Washing Delicates

- Turn garments inside out to reduce abrasion on creases and edges.

- Use the shortest wash cycle and lowest agitation setting available.

- Use mesh laundry bags for panty hose, lingerie and delicate blouses.

- Overdrying can cause static, pilling, progressive shrinkage, wrinkling, and puckered seams.

Use warm, not hot, settings to warm fabric and remove wrinkles.

Take clothes out of the dryer lightly damp and warm.

Shake well and hang to cool and air dry.

Tug gently on seams to stretch the thread and minimize puckering.

Dry Cleaning—the most for your money

- Always clean both parts of a two-piece garment together to avoid developing a color variation.

- Point out spots and stains to your cleaner, and identify the cause. Also identify the fiber content if the label is missing.

- Request that ID tags be attached to your garments with safety pins instead of staples.

- Remove delicate buttons or cover them tightly with aluminum foil to prevent damage from dry cleaning chemicals.

- Try bulk dry cleaning or "dry clean only" for items that don't require professional pressing. It can be a real money saver.

- Use one of the in-your-dryer cleaning products to extend the time between trips to the dry cleaner. Garments go into a big plastic bag with a chemical-infused sheet, and then tumble in the dryer for a specified time. Remove and hang immediately. Effectively removes wrinkles, body odor, smoke smell, and surface soil.

- Plastic cleaner bags hold heat and attract moisture. Remove the bags before you put garments into the closet. And while you're at it, swap the wire hanger for a more supportive one.

- Remember that most quality dry cleaners also offer clothing repair services, dyeing, water-repellency treatment, and other helpful services.

Pressing Matters

The right pressing equipment makes a big difference in the ease of the task and the finished appearance of the garment. You should have:

♦ **A good "shot-of-steam" iron** with a nonstick coating and visible water level indicator.

♦ **Well-padded ironing board.** Use cotton canvas covers; metallic ones cause heat to bounce back and can damage delicate fabrics.

♦ **A sleeve board* and pressing mitt*** make it easy to press sleeves without creases. They also help reach hard-to-press areas.

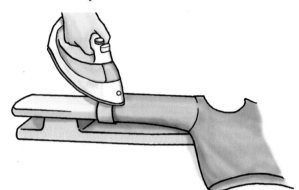

♦ **A seam roll*** allows you to prevent unsightly ridges when you press seams open after laundering or cleaning. Because the seam roll is rounded and the bottom of the iron is flat, the garment curves away from the iron so you press only the stitching line and not the edges of the seam allowance.

seam roll

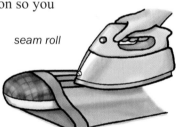

♦ **Cotton see-through pressing cloth*** prevents the fabric surface from getting shiny but still allows you to see what you're doing.

press cloth

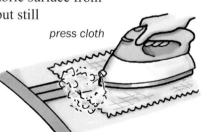

♦ **Hot iron cleaner*** keeps your soleplate clean and smooth. Use it on a hot iron with several layers of damp cloth, as directed.

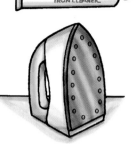

♦ **Soleplate cover*** makes it easy to press heat-sensitive synthetics without creating a shine. Remove it from your iron periodically to clear away any lint buildup and to clean the soleplate.

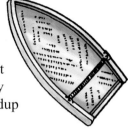

*Available in fabric stores

Pressing Pointers

♦ Always test iron temperature in a hidden area of the garment first. A too-hot iron can melt a hole in synthetic fabric.

♦ Press delicate fabrics on the wrong side or use a press cloth or soleplate cover for top pressing.

♦ Use a little spray starch or sizing to keep cotton, linen, or lace looking crisp.

♦ Allow garments to cool before you move them or the creases you just pressed will fall right out. Fabrics have "memory" only when they cool.

♦ Eliminate daily touch-up pressing by choosing tomorrow's outfit this evening and letting it hang outside the closet, where most wrinkles will fall out overnight.

♦ Use a portable steamer to gently freshen garments and remove wrinkles when crisp edges and creases are not required.

The Bottom Line — Shoes and Boots

Quality shoes and boots are an investment and deserve good care, and the same is true for handbags and portfolios.

♦ Spray fabric shoes with a stain guard before the first wearing, since they cannot readily be cleaned.

♦ Give leather shoes a paste polish before the first wearing, and future stains will penetrate less easily.

♦ Spray new suede shoes with a non-silicone finish to help repel water and stains.

♦ Use a soft mat under the pedals of your car to avoid scraping the back side of your heels.

♦ Rotate your shoes. Fine footwear will last longer if you allow it to rest between wearings.

♦ Store shoes with shoe trees to maintain the shape. Cedar shoe trees also absorb moisture and odors.

♦ Dry damp shoes away from any heat sources, which could cause the leather to crack.

♦ Clean leather shoes as needed with a special leather cleaner, or for heavier soil use saddle soap and water, rinsing thoroughly.

♦ Condition the newly cleaned leather with a lanolin-based leather conditioner to replenish the natural oils.

♦ Polish leather shoes with a cream or paste polish. Apply with a clean cloth, allow to dry, and buff with a polishing brush. Wax or liquid polish can dry out the leather and cause cracking.

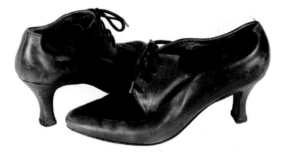

♦ Revive suede shoes by rubbing briskly with a stiff brush. Use a special eraser called a suede bar to remove dirt and stains.

♦ Rinse off damaging white salt marks immediately with a 50/50 mixture of white distilled vinegar and water. Wipe off excess moisture and dry away from heat.

♦ Have new heel tips put on heels as soon as the original ones begin to show wear.

♦ Consider resoling fine shoes if the uppers are in good condition. It's far less expensive than buying new ones.

Chapter 17
Custom Clothing

Hire a Professional Dressmaker

If you are hooked on the luxury of having exactly the color, style, fit and fabric you want, but don't have the time or the skill level to tackle a particular project, consider hiring a professional seamstress to make it for you. To locate a certified professional in your area, check out the Association of Sewing and Design Professionals at www.sewingprofessionals.org.

If You Sew...or Would Like To

Sewing enthusiasts have special advantages such as these when it comes to building effective wardrobes:

♦ When you need an exact color or specific figure-flattering style.

♦ When you need specialized fit for your unique shape.

♦ When you need an item not currently in season.

Whatever the need...YOU CAN SEW IT!! However, with all those advantages, there are some typical wardrobing weaknesses many of us sewing enthusiasts seem to share. Do any of these describe you?

1. **Overlooking ourselves.** We can get so excited about a particularly interesting fabric combination or intricate pattern detail that we leap right into a project without ever considering how the finished garment will suit US.

    If that sounds like you, review the first six chapters to fine-tune your awareness of the points of connection you can create between your physical characteristics and your wardrobe choices.

2. **Getting "over-printy."** Let's face it...prints, plaids and textured fabrics are much more enticing on the bolt than a plain solid. But those solids make up the workhorse items in any wardrobe.

    Too many prints equals too few wardrobe combinations. Discipline yourself to sew more solids for a more versatile wardrobe.

3. **Doting on details.** An intricately styled jacket with detailed seaming, contrasting piping, buttons and trims may show off your sewing abilities, but

it probably won't mix as well in your wardrobe as a more streamlined style.

As a rule, simple styles sewn in fabulous fabrics will give you the best return on your sewing time investment.

4. **Under-accessorizing.** Since sewing enthusiasts spend more shopping time in fabric stores than in department stores, we often miss the message that accessories are necessary to complete any fashion look. Review Chapter 12 carefully to absorb this important wardrobe lesson.

5. **Becoming TOO thrifty.** There's nothing wrong with appreciating the savings sewing offers when compared with fine quality ready-mades. But fight the tendency to become downright CHEAP. Treat yourself to the very finest fabrics you can afford. They will cooperate with you in the construction process. And they'll last for years in your wardrobe.

6. **Believing you have to sew EVERYTHING in your wardrobe.** Even industry professionals recognize that today's busy lifestyles make it impossible to sew everything you wear. Sew the things that bring you joy in the creative process, and don't feel a smidgen of guilt about buying the other items you need.

To Sew or Buy?

It Makes Sense to Sew...

1. When you can't find what you want in ready-to-wear. Choosing your own combination of fabric and pattern vastly increases your options.

2. When you can make the item in less time than it would take you to shop for it.

3. When you're capable of creating better quality clothing than you could afford ready-made.

4. When your body proportions make it difficult to find a good fit in a ready-made garment.

5. When you find expensive items that would be easy to copy.

6. When you can create a big impact by sewing simple styles in smashing fabrics.

It Makes Sense to Buy...

1. When your time is worth more than the money saved by making the garment.

2. When you don't have time to make what you need.

3. When the details or the fabric are beyond your skills.

4. When the color, fit and styling are great for you and so is the price.

5. When you find a great item at a great price—even if it needs minor adjustments in fit or detail. With basic sewing skills, you can easily upgrade a bargain by:

   • replacing average buttons with distinctive ones.
   • adding a fashionable belt.
   • redoing poorly stitched hems.
   • changing the length for a better proportion.
   • adding or replacing trims.
   • adding or removing shoulder pads for smoother fit.
   • tapering side seams for closer-to-the-body fit.

Organize Your Fabric Stash

Many sewing enthusiasts have discovered that, even when they can't find time to sew, there's always time to buy more fabric. But before you buy one more yard, you need to beg, borrow or steal some time to organize your current fabric stash. Goodness knows what treasures you may find in the process.

Clean House

Do a clean-out of your stash just as you did with the clothes in your closet.

♦ Check color first. If it's not in your color fan, discard it. Or if you're adventurous, try dyeing it a more flattering color. You can generally dye a cool color to a warmer version, but to dye a warm color to a cool one you must also go to a darker value. For more ideas, see page 191.

♦ Tastes change. If you no longer love it, let it go.

♦ Evaluate prints carefully. Because they are so attention-getting, they need to be absolutely right for you. See page 36-37 for a complete discussion of print selection.

♦ Consider the weight of the fabric. Bulky or heavily textured fabrics add visual pounds. Discard any that don't meet your style objectives.

Dispose of Your Discards Immediately

♦ Have a swap meet with your sewing friends. Your discard could be the fabric of their dreams, and vice versa.

♦ Include the discards in a garage sale.

♦ Give it away. Many charities are grateful recipients of fabrics, and it's a tax deduction for you.

Catalog What's Left

Here's one easy system:

1. Glue a swatch of each piece to its own 3x5 card. Include swatches of fabrics you've already sewn if the garment is still in your closet.

2. Record the fiber content, width, yardage, care instructions, storage location, and any other information you want.

Fabric name _____

attach swatch here

Fiber content _____

Width _____ Yardage _____

Care Instruction _____

Storage Location _____

---

3. Store all the cards in a zip-top bag, organized in any order that makes sense for you:
   • By color
   • By fabric type
   • By season
   • By end use
   • By fiber content
   • By weight (top/bottom)

We've also seen systems with swatches in clear plastic credit card holders, in photo-sleeve pages in a 3-ring binder, and on an oversized safety pin with sticky labels. Use whatever works for you.

Now Use Your System

♦ Use your file as a guide for planning new projects so they will blend with what you already have.

♦ Take the file along any time you shop—especially when you travel to a sewing expo.

♦ Select your next sewing project by comparing your file pages with your current wardrobe and finding new coordination possibilities.

Store Your Stash Efficiently

♦ Preshrink fabrics before you put them away. Clip one corner diagonally to indicate that the piece is preshrunk.

♦ Designate a fabric closet. Add floor to ceiling shelves and store folded fabric by color, weight or end use.

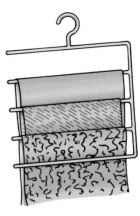

♦ Or fold each piece over a tubular hanger and hang from a conventional closet rod.

♦ Roll, rather than fold, very crisp or deep pile fabrics to avoid creases. Ask your fabric store for empty cardboard tubes.

♦ Organize your interfacings:

• Discard any old unidentified fusibles.
• Stock up on your favorites so you'll always have some on hand. Larger pieces will cut to better advantage too.
• Try the Palmer/Pletsch line of PerfectFuse interfacings. Thorough instructions are included in the packages.

♦ What about scraps?

• Toss anything that's too small to use, keeping only enough for some future repair of the garment.
• Roll the keepers and store in a large box sorted by color or on hangers.

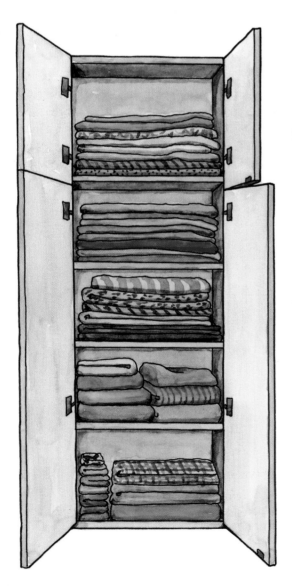

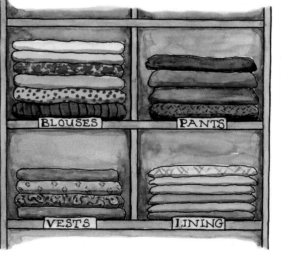

roll scraps and store sorted by color

store trims on cardboard rolls

store fabric sorted by end use

Store Patterns Efficiently

♦ Keep the pattern pieces and the original envelope in a large zip-top bag.

♦ Or store pattern pieces in a large manila envelope and glue the pattern envelope to the outside.

♦ Store patterns by garment type in a file cabinet or storage box.

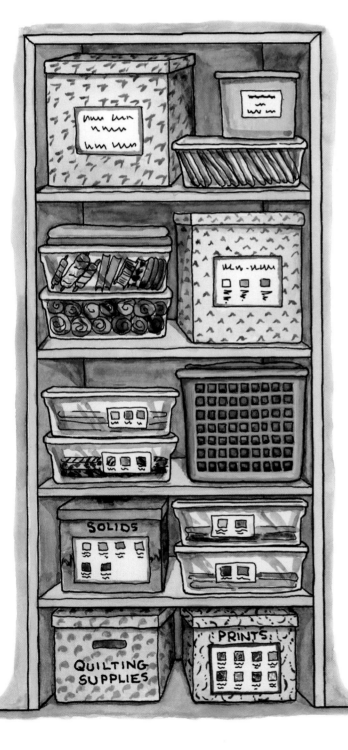

Shopping for Fabric Capsules

Plan ahead for wardrobe versatility by selecting your fabric in groupings, with a capsule of coordinating garments in mind. This capsule concept is far easier to execute in a fabric store than in a clothing boutique where you might find the right colors and fabric, but made into the wrong styles or sizes for you.

1. Select a top-quality bottom-weight fabric in a favorite solid from your color fan—maybe your key neutral—for matching jacket, skirt and pants.

2. Carry that bolt around the store to find a closely matched top-weight for a shirt, blouse or knit top to complete your core four (page 97).

3. Seek out coordinating top-weights for accent blouses and jackets.

4. Look for bottom-weights to match at least a few of your accent top fabrics so you can create additional color columns.

5. Pick one or two prints that repeat the various solid colors you've chosen.

6. Spread out all the possibilities and mix and match them until you narrow the selection to the pieces you'll need for your capsule. Don't forget to compare them with your swatch file of on-hand fabrics. If you're consistently shopping in your best colors, you'll almost certainly find additional combinations there.

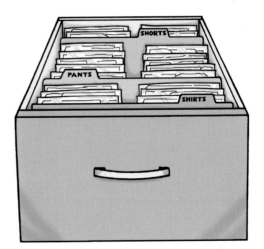

For additional organization ideas see the Palmer/Pletsch book *Dream Sewing Spaces*.

7. Buy the new fabric all at once to avoid disappointment later and guard against changing seasonal color trends. Of course you don't have to sew it all right away. But remember that choosing simple pattern styles will showcase those beautiful fabrics and speed your construction time as well.

8. If you don't have specific patterns selected yet for each garment, use these guidelines for amounts to buy for sizes up to about 14:

YARDAGE GUIDE	45" Fabric	54-60" Fabric
Slim skirt	2x finished length plus 8" for hem, waistband	finished length plus 6"
Fuller skirt	same	same
Pants	same	same
Long-sleeve blouse	2 1/4 yards	1 1/2 yards
Shell blouse	1 yard	1 yard
Hip-length jacket	3 yards	2 yards

Smart Shopping in Pattern Catalogs

♦ You can look at all major brands online to see trends. Or you can look at catalogs in fabric stores. If you see similar styles in several catalogs, compare line drawings.

♦ Carefully study the front photo pages of each catalog for the season's newest directions in color, styles, wardrobe coordination, and accessories. When you spot a look you like, you can find the pattern in the body of the catalog by checking the index of style numbers on the very last page of the book.

♦ The hundreds of designs in each catalog are grouped by category, with the newest designs photographed in the introductory pages and placed near the front in their respective sections.

♦ To make room for new styles added each season, slow-sellers are discontinued.

♦ Patterns labeled "easy" contain fewer pieces and simplified instructions. But any pattern can be fast to sew if it has these details:

• Gathers or easing instead of darts or pleats.

• Few details like plackets, yokes or topstitching.

• Neckline finishes like binding or facing instead of a collar.

• No pieces cut on the bias grain line.

♦ The small line drawings show to-scale proportions, design details, and seam lines. They are often more enlightening than the fashion illustrations or photographs of the same garments. Consider carefully how those lines will look on your body. What areas will the lines emphasize?

♦ You may want to open the envelope and study the drawings of the pattern pieces on the guide sheet to understand details of the design and how the garment is constructed.

♦ Suggested fabrics are those most suitable for this design.

• A pattern labeled "knits only" requires the fabric's stretch to provide ease for a comfortable, flattering fit.

• A pattern labeled "not suitable for plaid" includes pattern shapes that prevent the plaid lines from matching at major seams.

♦ You'll need the "with nap" yardage amount if your fabric has any one-directional characteristic like a pile surface or a print with all motifs headed the same way.

♦ These icons on a pattern catalog page or pattern envelope indicate that the style can be sewn to fit that body type with minimum alterations. That isn't quite the same thing as saying that it will flatter that body shape.

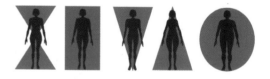

The Pattern Envelope

♦ The envelope front shows the various views included in the pattern. Fashion sketches drawn on an idealized body don't provide much insight into true garment proportions, but they do offer wardrobe coordination possibilities and accessorizing ideas.

♦ Line drawings on the back of the envelope (or on the guide sheet inside) show the true proportions and design details.

♦ Finished garment lengths are printed on the tissue, so check those before trimming to your size. They help you know how much fullness to expect by answering questions like "how full is the skirt?" or "how wide is the pant leg?" Compare these measurements with garments you already know are flattering.

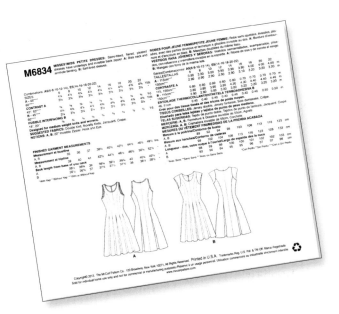

♦ Garment descriptions give you information about fit and details that may not be obvious from the pictures.

♦ Patterns are made to body measurements plus standard wearing ease (breathing room). Most patterns also include design ease—extra fabric to create the intended fashion look. The terms shown here—fitted, semifitted, loose fitting, very loose fitting—are used to indicate the amount of design ease in a pattern, and the drawings at right are examples of those descriptive terms.

Fitted	semifitted	loose fitting	very loose

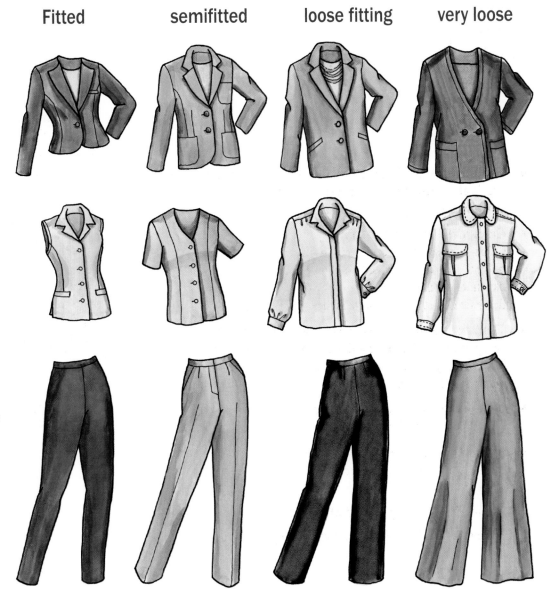

Creative Combinations

Successfully combining patterns and fabrics is the most creative part of sewing. It can also be the most challenging. You can use either the pattern or the fabric as your starting point.

Starting With the Pattern

When you have an itemized list of wardrobe needs, select the patterns first. You can look for specific styling and details, and then find the right fabric to execute the design. You have more freedom in style choices when you aren't limited by the characteristics of a fabric you've already purchased.

The following steps will help you find the ideal fabric for your pattern:

1. Check the list of suggested fabrics on the pattern envelope. The sketches or photographs of the style are additional clues.

    - Is it shown in a solid or a print?

    - Does the style need a soft fabric to fall gracefully or a crisp one to hold a defined shape?

    - Look at similar styles in department stores or clothing catalogs for additional fabric clues.

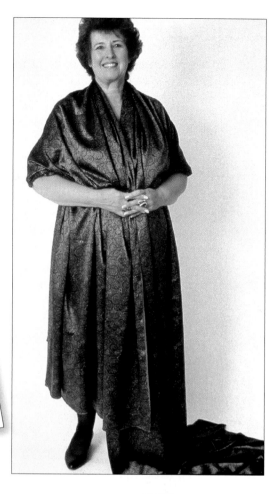

2. If some of the suggested fabrics aren't available, substitute other fabrics with weight and drape similar to those listed.

3. Preview the finished garment by draping the fabric on your body to simulate the design while you stand in front of a full-length mirror.

    - If the design has gathers, gather the fabric with your hands and evaluate the bulk and the drape.

    - Do the gathers fall softly or stand away from your body?

    - Would the fabric drape better on the bias?

    - Do layers of overlap (jacket front with facings, wrap skirt, etc.) become too bulky?

    - Does the fabric pattern or texture add unwanted body bulk, physically or visually?

This DVD is excellent for helping you understand whether a fabric will work for your design: www.palmerpletsch.com

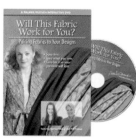

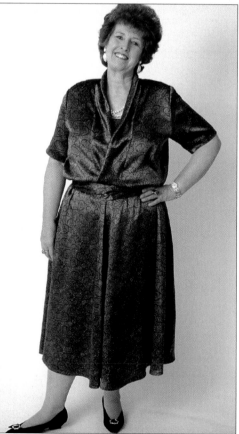

Starting With Fabric

- If you are selecting a pattern to use with a print or plaid fabric you've already purchased, be sure there are no restrictions for those fabrics on the back of the envelope.

  - Almost any style will work with a small allover print, but large prints usually require relatively simple styles. Most design details will seem to disappear into a print fabric.

  - One-way designs and prints with obvious motifs look best when they can be matched at major seam lines. Be sure you have enough extra yardage to accommodate a modified layout.

- Crisp fabrics lend themselves to tailored styles with darts and seams to shape them to body contours.

- Soft, lightweight, fluid fabrics work best in designs with few details and more fullness and drape.

- The softer and more drapable the fabric, the more fullness you can use in the design without getting a bulky look. A gathered skirt that would work beautifully in challis would be bulky and awkward in corduroy, for example.

- Solid fabrics can spotlight interesting seaming and design details. Construction details show to best advantage in relatively firm fabrics like flannel, gabardine, brushed twill, raw silk and linen. Soft fabrics can show off gathering.

- Sheer fabrics require simple designs, few seams and limited details—ideally with narrow hems and with binding instead of traditional facings.

- Pile fabrics like velveteen and corduroy are easiest to sew in styles with minimum detailing.

- Use a border across a shoulder area and the associated sleeve cap to create a strong horizontal emphasis.

- Be careful about placing a border along a slim skirt's hem; the horizontal low on the body can make the figure appear shorter and heavier.

- It isn't possible to use a border at the hem of an A-line or gored skirt because the lower edge of the pattern piece is curved.

- Border prints and embroideries limit pattern choice, but with creativity the results can be exciting.

  - Seam blouses at center front, creating a double border. Repeat on the center front of the matching skirt.

  - Asymmetrical vertical placement of a border creates a flattering, lengthening effect.

  - Place a narrow embroidered or eyelet edge at hem, sleeve edge and collar.

  - Use a border vertically to jazz up a simple vest.

Using border prints strategically can bring attention up toward the face.

Check Your Choices

If you can answer "Yes" to most of these questions, you have planned a wardrobe winner. If not, perhaps your plan needs to be modified.

- ☐ Does this project fill a need in my wardrobe? Impulse purchases usually aren't a wise use of your dollars or your time.

- ☐ Is the color one of my personal best?

- ☐ Will this item work with at least three things in my existing wardrobe? If not, have I planned additional coordinates to sew?

- ☐ Do I own the necessary accessories to complete the look? If not, am I willing to purchase them?

- ☐ If I've worn this fiber before, was it comfortable for me?

- ☐ Am I willing to care for this fabric as the manufacturer recommends?

- ☐ Are the print and/or texture flattering to me?

- ☐ Do the lines of the pattern enhance my figure assets and divert attention from my challenge areas?

- ☐ Are the construction details within the range of my sewing skills?

- ☐ If I have worn a similar style before, was it comfortable and flattering?

- ☐ Is it either a classic style or on the upswing of the fashion curve so I can wear it long enough to get full value for my investment?

- ☐ Does the total cost plus the sewing time required fit my time/money budget?

Be Your Own Designer

You can get great mileage by using a favorite pattern again and again. You have already perfected the fit and become familiar with the construction sequence. You know the style looks good and feels comfortable on your body. And you can individualize each garment with distinctive fabric choices and new fashion details.

Sewing is easier the second time around if you record the following information on the guide sheet:

- ◆ Date sewn
- ◆ Weight and body measurements
- ◆ Alterations made to pattern
- ◆ Fabric and interfacing used

Worth Repeating

Vary the look of a repeat-performance pattern by choosing fabrics with an entirely different mood.

- ◆ Summer print skirt and shell, linen jacket
- ◆ Velveteen skirt and cardigan, lace shell
- ◆ Wool skirt, silk crepe shell, tweed jacket.

basic shell

slim skirt

cardigan jacket

Individualize a basic blazer with details like these:

♦ Round the lapels and collar edges. Use a French curve for consistent shaping.

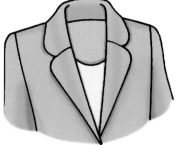

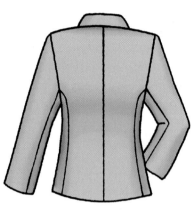

French curve

♦ Eliminate back and sleeve vents for a dressier look.

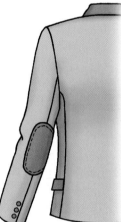

♦ Add elbow patches and sew the pocket flaps and upper collar from coordinating suede or suede-look fabric.

♦ Add (or eliminate) patch pockets.

♦ Topstitch narrow ribbon or braid trim to the collar, lapel or sleeve edges before constructing the garment.

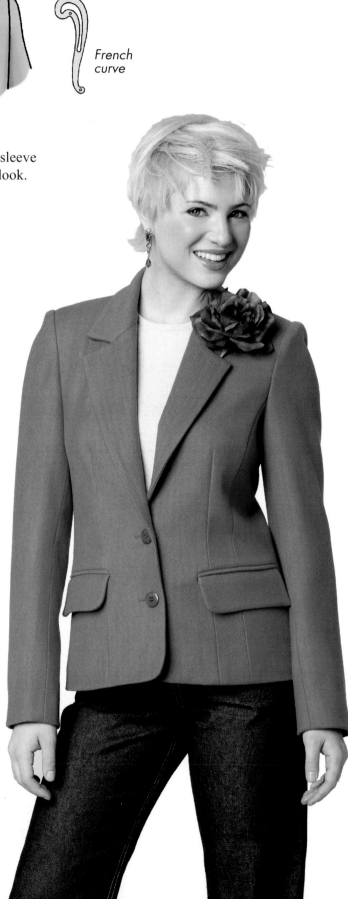

Customize a Blouse Pattern

You can sew a whole wardrobe of blouses from one pattern with customized details like these:

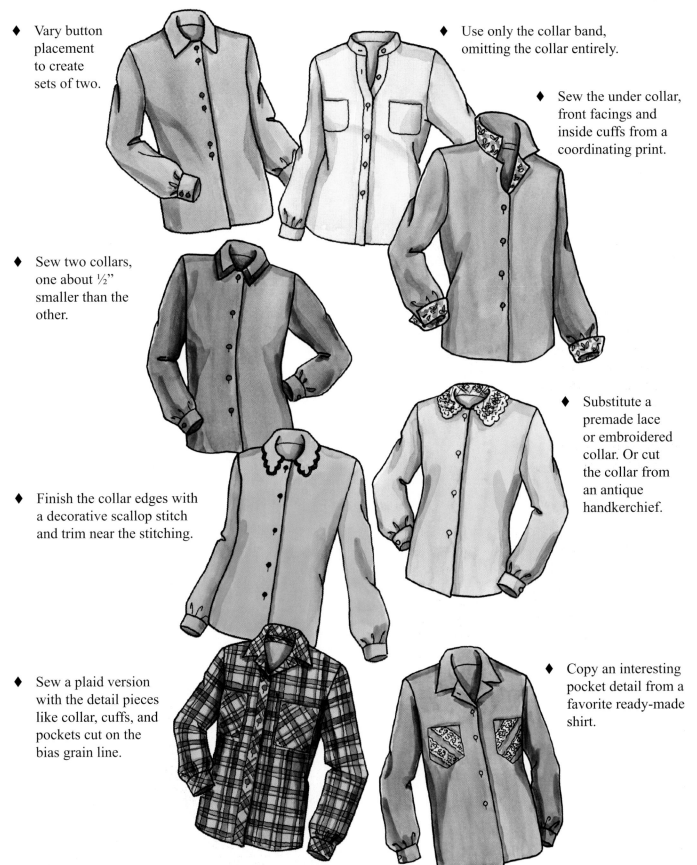

♦ Vary button placement to create sets of two.

♦ Use only the collar band, omitting the collar entirely.

♦ Sew the under collar, front facings and inside cuffs from a coordinating print.

♦ Sew two collars, one about ½" smaller than the other.

♦ Substitute a premade lace or embroidered collar. Or cut the collar from an antique handkerchief.

♦ Finish the collar edges with a decorative scallop stitch and trim near the stitching.

♦ Sew a plaid version with the detail pieces like collar, cuffs, and pockets cut on the bias grain line.

♦ Copy an interesting pocket detail from a favorite ready-made shirt.

Chapter 18
Fashion Updates

A magnetic pin catcher such as a Grabbit, with a wide, shallow surface to hold lots of pins. Turn it over to pick up spilled pins too.

On page 88 we introduced the idea of updating garments from your closet to be more contemporary or more flattering. Even a novice sewer can handle minor updates. Start by collecting the basic equipment:

The Basic Necessities

♦ Sharp 8" dressmaker shears

♦ Sharp embroidery scissors

♦ Hand needles, size 10 sharps for hems

♦ Round head pins

And you certainly will appreciate the handy extras shown here.

Seam ripper

Pinch-and-pull bodkin—great for replacing elastic

Fray Check liquid ravel preventer. Run a thin coating along a fabric edge for a permanent seam finish. Stop runs in nylons too.

Measuring tools—tape measure, yardstick, sewing gauge

Basting tape—narrow double-stick tape that replaces hand basting. Great for zippers, matching plaids.

Erasable fabric markers in light or dark color. Some erase with a damp cloth, others disappear on their own in 24-48 hours.

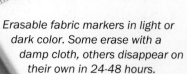

Flat skirt hooks in black and silver

Makeover Ideas

Color Update: Dyeing

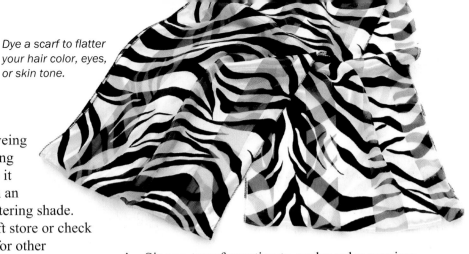

Dye a scarf to flatter your hair color, eyes, or skin tone.

If you're the do-it-yourself type, dyeing can be an almost free method of updating your wardrobe to your new colors. Use it to refresh a faded garment or transform an unflattering colored item to a more flattering shade.

Purchase RIT dye at your local craft store or check art supply stores and online resources for other options. Liquid dyes are easiest to use because the color particles are already dissolved and blended. Follow package instructions carefully.

Use dye on washable garments to:

- Return washable black or other dark-colored garments to their original depth of color.

- Transform light-wash or faded jeans to a more slimming, polished dark-wash look.

- Warm up a cool garment color. A pale yellow or camel dye will transform pinks to peaches, blues to aquas, mint greens to yellow-greens, and so on.

- Cool down a warm-color garment by covering the original color with a darker version of the same family. You could convert an aqua blue to royal blue or navy, for example. Since you can't pull the existing warm (golden) tones out of the color, you'll have to cover them up instead.

- Transform a print garment. The dye will affect all the colors similarly, so a pale yellow or camel dye can warm up a cool-tone print and the motifs remain clearly visible.

- Since a transformation to cooler color requires going darker too, it is much tougher to dye a print from warm to cool without obscuring the motifs.

- Tone down a too-contrasting print or plaid or check—especially black and white combinations, which are too strong to flatter most people. The white area will accept dye in the color of your choice while the black areas will be unaffected. If the print garment is a skirt or pant, consider dyeing a plain white blouse or T-shirt in the same dye bath to create a coordinated outfit.

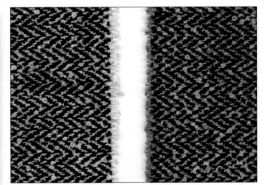

The original cool blue, below, has been warmed up.

Warm up a black and white tweed wool.

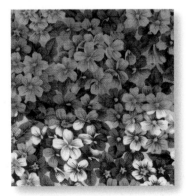

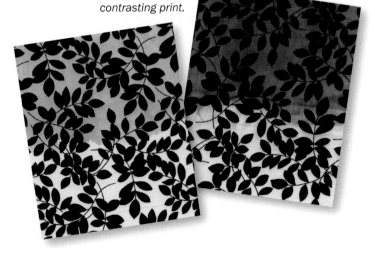

Tone down a too-contrasting print.

191

Better Buttons

This easiest of updates can have a surprisingly big impact. Consider these changes:

♦ Trade white plastic shirt buttons for classier mother-of-pearl ones.

♦ Replace faded buttons with fresh ones that match the garment's color accurately.

♦ Swap bright metal buttons for more subtle burnished or antiqued ones.

♦ Change to buttons that repeat a personal color element—typically your hair color—within the garment. Brass, pewter and tortoiseshell buttons can create this effect easily.

♦ Connect buttons to your facial structure, adopting square or triangular buttons if your features are angular, for example.

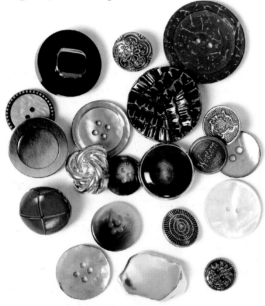

Perfect Hems

The right hem or sleeve length can make the difference between dowdy and dynamite. Changes of even ½" can have a big impact.

To Redo a Garment Hem:

1. Carefully remove the existing stitches with a seam ripper or small scissors. Press out the original hemline crease.

2. Try on the garment and have a friend mark the desired new length, measuring up from the floor an even distance all around.

3. Fold up the hem on the marked line and lightly press the new hem crease.

4. Cut away excess width of fabric. In most garments the hem depth should be between 1½" and 2"— slightly narrower in heavier fabrics, slightly wider in lighter weights.

5. Trim seam allowances within the hem area to ¼".

6. Finish the edge of the hem with one these ways:

 • Pinking shears

 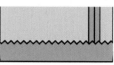

 • Zigzag machine stitch

 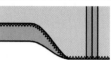

 • Seam tape

 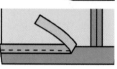

 • Serger stitch

7. Use the hand blind stitch, which never leaves a ridge on the outside of the garment.

 • Size 10 sharp needles ("sharps" are a type of needle, not just an indication that they aren't dull) let you catch only a fiber or two of the outside fabric for an invisible hem.

 • A single strand of polyester thread provides the strongest, longest-lasting stitches.

 • Fold down ¼" of the hem edge and stitch between the two layers. Use a loose running stitch about ½" long, catching only a fiber of the outside fabric. Pull on the fabric every six inches to loosen the stitches and make a small knot in the hem allowance to strengthen the hem.

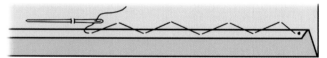

 • These instructions assume a straight hem edge. A curved edge will require an easing stitch along the cut edge to shape the hem flat against the garment. If the side seams are tapered, you will need to restitch them to angle outward within the hem area to make the hem edge match the skirt width.

Other Ways to Shorten

Use Tucks

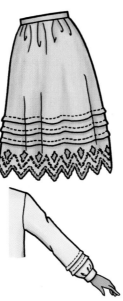

This is the easiest way to shorten a lightweight skirt with a narrow border print or decorative hem detail. And it is a far easier way to shorten a shirt sleeve than removing and replacing the cuff or shortening from the sleeve cap. Use this technique on garments cut from straight fabric panels, but not flared or A-shaped ones. A series of several small tucks makes a more attractive detail than a single large one.

1. Determine how much you need to shorten the garment. Determine how many tucks you'll need and divide the total distance by the number of tucks to determine the depth of each tuck you'll sew.

2. Mark tuck stitching lines with a water-erasable marker. Use a sewing gauge to maintain an even spacing.

3. Fold the fabric along each marked line in turn, pinning or basting along the stitching line. Remember that stitching ½" from the fold takes up 1" of garment length.

4. Try on the garment to double-check the adjusted length.

5. Stitch the tucks with a medium-length straight stitch, overlapping the ends of the stitching about ½" to secure.

6. Remove the pins or basting and lightly press the tucks toward the hem or cuff.

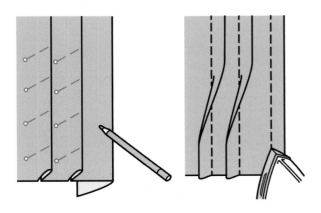

Shorten From the Top

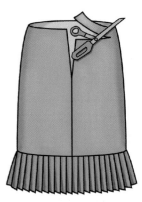

This is ideal for garments with wider decorative hem details because it doesn't disturb the bottom edge. It also works well when you want a little more room in the waistband.

1. Remove the button or hook and eye, the waistband and zipper.

2. Cut away from the top the amount you want to remove from the garment's length. You don't need to add back a waistline seam allowance; it's already there.

3. Lengthen any darts or change them to soft gathers. If the original skirt was gathered, replace the gathering stitches at the new upper edge.

4. Replace the zipper.

5. Reattach the waistband, gathering or easing the skirt edge to fit. To make the waist larger, simply allow less of the waistband ends to overlap.

6. Replace the button or hook and eye closure.

Lengthening

While the amount you can shorten a garment is almost unlimited, you can lengthen only by as much as the width of the original hem.

1. Carefully remove the original hem and press out the crease.

2. For stubborn creases, try using a press cloth dampened with a mixture of half water and half vinegar. The vinegar helps unset the old crease.

3. Mark the new length and lightly press the new crease.

4. Use a hand blind stitch to invisibly secure the hem, as described on the previous page.

5. Lightly press the finished hem.

6. If the original crease still shows, add several parallel rows of topstitching to camouflage it.

If you need to lengthen so much that the remaining hem allowance is less than an inch, add a facing to the cut edge.

1. Remove the old hem, mark the new length, and lightly press.

2. Cut a straight-grain strip of color-matched lining fabric as long as the circumference of the hem plus ½". Make the strip 2½" wide minus the width of garment hem you have remaining.

3. Join the ends of the lining strip with a ¼" seam and press open. Finish one long edge of the strip with one of the methods from the hemming how-tos on page 192.

4. Match the strip with the cut edge of the garment hem, right sides together. Join with a ¼" seam.

5. Use a hand blind stitch to invisibly secure the hem.

6. Lightly press the finished hem at the lower edge.

For Too-Short Pants

If you don't have enough hem allowance to lengthen the pants, consider restyling them instead.

♦ Shorten casual or slim pants to mid-calf length for capris.

♦ Shorten to knee length for city shorts, with or without cuffs.

♦ Shorten fuller pants to below-the-knee length for gauchos.

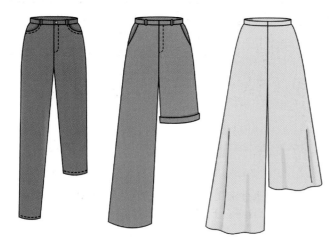

Restyling Culottes

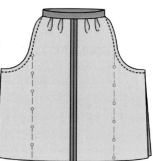

Turn full pants or culottes into a slim skirt.

1. Carefully remove the hem and unstitch the inside leg seam with a seam ripper or small scissors.

2. Mark new seam lines at center front and center back with a yardstick and water-erasable marker. Follow the grain line straight down from just above the crotch curve.

3. Baste the marked seam and try on the garment. Make any necessary adjustments.

4. Trim away the excess fabric 5/8" beyond the basting and stitch a permanent seam.

5. Press the seam allowances open. Restitch the hem.

Tapering

Ramp up the figure flattery of a straight skirt or fuller pant by tapering the garment slightly from hip to hemline. This technique can't be successfully applied to A-line skirts because the waist and hem edges are cut on a curve.

1. Carefully unstitch the hem.

2. Pin or baste new side seams, starting just below the fullest point of the hip and tapering toward the hemline.

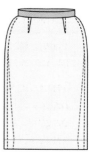

3. Try on the garment to determine if you want to taper it more or less, and adjust the pin positions accordingly.

4. On pants, you may want to taper a smaller amount on the outside leg seam and taper the inside leg seam as well for a more balanced look.

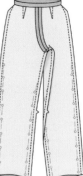

5. Stitch the new seams, tapering back outward at the same angle within the hem allowance.

6. Trim the seam allowances to 5/8", remove the remainder of the original stitching, and press seam allowances open.

7. Restitch the original hem. Press.

Tapering Sleeves

Manufacturers and pattern makers often make sleeves fuller than necessary, which gives the impression of unwanted body bulk. This is especially common in sizes above 12 or 14.

Fortunately, it is relatively easy to narrow the sleeve, allowing visual space between the arms and the torso.

1. Unstitch the lining, if any, and the sleeve hem.

2. Turn the sleeve wrong side out and baste a new seam line, tapering from the armhole to the wrist. If the sleeve has two seams, you can distribute the amount of taper between them, or choose the one that doesn't have any placket detail to complicate the process.

3. Try on the garment to determine if you want more or less shaping and make any necessary adjustments.

4. Stitch the new seams, tapering back outward at the same angle within the hem allowance.

5. Stitch a corresponding tapered seam in the lining if necessary.

6. Trim the seam allowances to 5/8", remove the remainder of the original stitching and press seam allowances open. A seam roll (see page 176) makes the pressing much easier.

7. Restitch the original hem, or a shorter one if necessary. Press.

8 Reattach the lining edge if necessary.

Instant Tapering

Hand or machine stitch an inverted pleat at the bottom of a pant leg or straight sleeve for a skinny look.

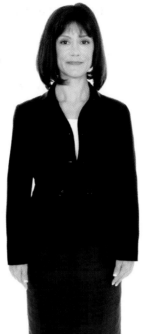

Make More Room

When an armhole is too snug, you can make it more comfortable by stitching the underarm seam ¼" deeper. Do not extend this deeper seam up into the sleeve cap or you will narrow the garment's shoulder line, making the armhole more snug rather than less.

Trim the seam allowance to ¼". Try on the garment and repeat the alteration if still more room is required.

Pants that are too snug in the crotch can be altered in the same way. Stitch only the curved area ¼" deeper, trim and try on. Repeat if more room is needed.

For more room in the seat only, stitch only the back half of the crotch curve lower. You probably need this alteration if the waistband rides low in the back or if you see fabric bunched up at the top of the leg, below your rear end.

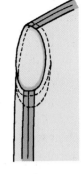

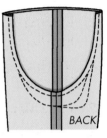

BACK

Shoulder Pads

Although the fashion trends for exaggerated shoulder lines come and go, lightweight shoulder support can match the angle of your shoulder to the shape of the garment and eliminate unsightly wrinkles and downward drag lines.

A slightly increased shoulder line also gives visual balance to fuller bust, hips, tummy or upper arms. And you won't look like a fullback. We promise.

♦ Add shoulder pads if you have wrinkles like this:

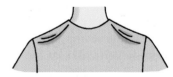

♦ Remove or reduce shoulder pads if you have wrinkles like this:

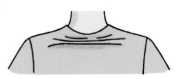

♦ Try on the garment and adjust the pads to the proper position, extending about ¼" into the sleeve cap. Pin from the outside of the garment.

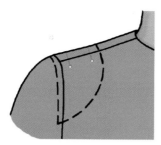

♦ From the inside, loosely hand stitch the pad to the seam allowance at the shoulder and the armhole.

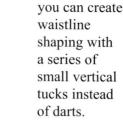

♦ If you don't want a shoulder pad permanently attached to the garment—either because it could curl in washing or because you sometimes wear the garment under a jacket with its own padding—use the removable foam shoulder pads that rest directly on your body and are held in place by the weight of the garment. Be sure to choose foam pads with an unglazed surface. Their slightly textural finish causes them to cling to the garment fabric and stay securely in place all day. (See Invisible Accesories, page 135.)

Reshape a Jacket or Blouse

The degree of waistline shaping in a blouse, jacket or dress should match the degree of waistline curve in your body.

♦ If a garment is cut too straight, you can often correct the problem by stitching a slight curve at the side seams and adding vertical darts to the side front and side back areas. Pin or baste these adjustments before stitching them permanently.

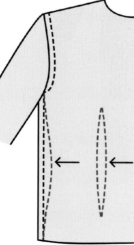

♦ In soft fabrics, you can create waistline shaping with a series of small vertical tucks instead of darts.

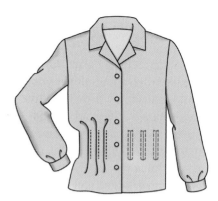

♦ If a garment is too shaped at the waist, you can often create a straighter silhouette just by carefully removing the stitching from any darts to release extra fullness.

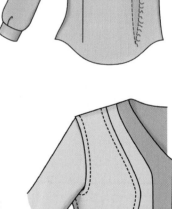

♦ If the excess shaping comes from princess seams, you can make new straighter stitching lines, but only to the extent that the garment has seam allowances wide enough to accommodate them.

Pati's Jacket Goes to Rosie

A closet purge often turns up some items that aren't great for you, but are too treasured to just donate to charity. Passing them along to a good friend can be a satisfying alternative.

Pati couldn't resist this creative jacket—a designer original she found at an art show. But when she updated her closet, she acknowledged that the intense, cool colors and the angularity of the design don't really flatter her. Fortunately, the jacket was perfect for her friend Rosie.

Just one problem: it was seriously too large. The solution was moderately complex:

1. Removed the sleeves, which were too long and needed to be shortened anyway.

2. Stitched new side seams and sleeve seams 1" deeper than the original. That made the sleeves 2" narrower and the garment 4" smaller in circumference (there are two side seams).

3. Re-cut the armhole to narrow the shoulder line and adjust for the deeper side seams.

4. Re-cut the sleeve cap to make the sleeve shorter and fit the new armhole.

5. Re-attached the sleeves.

6. Replaced the dated, thick shoulder pads with smaller ones.

Even if the new owner had to hire a professional to handle the restyling, the artistry and cost of the jacket justify the expense.

The end result—two happy women and one great garment saved.

NOTE: Yes, we also restyled Rosie's hair. See page 152 for details.

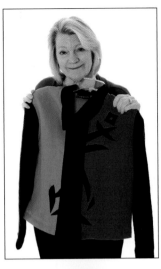

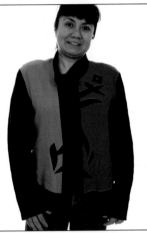

the jacket before alteration

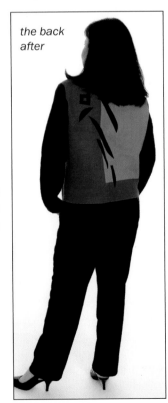

the back after

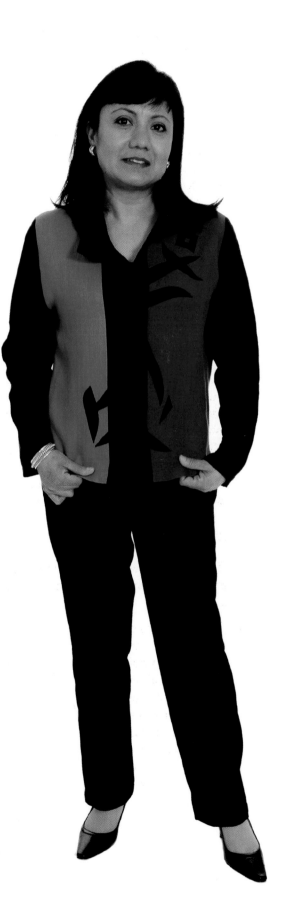

Chapter 19
Looking Good on the Go

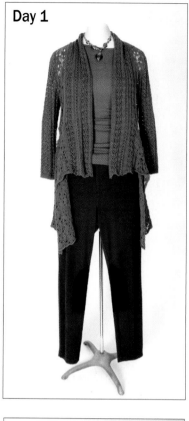

Day 1

Cartoon images of women traveling with piles of overstuffed suitcases are seriously out of date. Women today travel around the world for business and pleasure, and don't want to be burdened with excess luggage. But they do want to look good during their travels.

A few basic pieces can mix and match to create a week's worth of outfits, whether the look needs to be professional or casual. When you have built your wardrobe in capsule groupings (see Chapter 11), you will already have the right pieces hanging in your closet.

Our example illustrates a combined business and sightseeing trip—seven days of stylish outfits you can pack in a single carry-on bag. The same concept works equally well for a purely business trip or for more casual travel. Simply substitute garment styles and fabrics suited to those activities.

♦ **Start with three bottoms:**
  - Brown ponte knit legging
  - Brown skirt
  - Camel pant

♦ **Add matching or coordinating solid tops:**
  - Brown sweater shell
  - Beige turtleneck sweater
  - Teal knit shirt

♦ **Add two jackets suited to the climate of your destination:**
  - Ecru swing jacket
  - Zip-front camel jacket

♦ **Finish the grouping with a print top and solid sweater set:**
  - Houndstooth print top
  - Plum knit shell and lacy cardigan.

♦ **Include an assortment of scarves, jewelry and a pashmina** to adapt the basic garments for more/less casual activities and for temperature variations.

Here's how you might mix the example pieces for a 7-day trip:

Day 1 – Brown leggings, plum knit shell, and matching cardigan make a comfy outfit for the plane.

Day 2 – Camel pant and matching jacket over teal knit shirt, with pashmina.

Day 3 – Brown skirt, beige turtleneck, and camel jacket. Replace the jacket with the pashmina for dressier dinner evening.

Day 4 – Brown legging, brown sweater shell, and plum cardigan. Plum print scarf links the colors.

Day 5 – Camel pant, teal knit shirt, and ecru swing jacket—pashmina optional.

Day 6 – Brown skirt, beige turtleneck, ecru swing jacket with animal-print scarf.

Day 7 – Brown legging, print top, and camel zipper jacket.

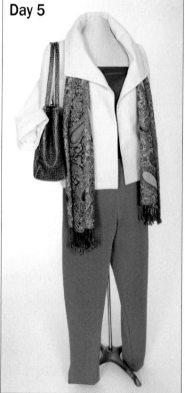

Day 5

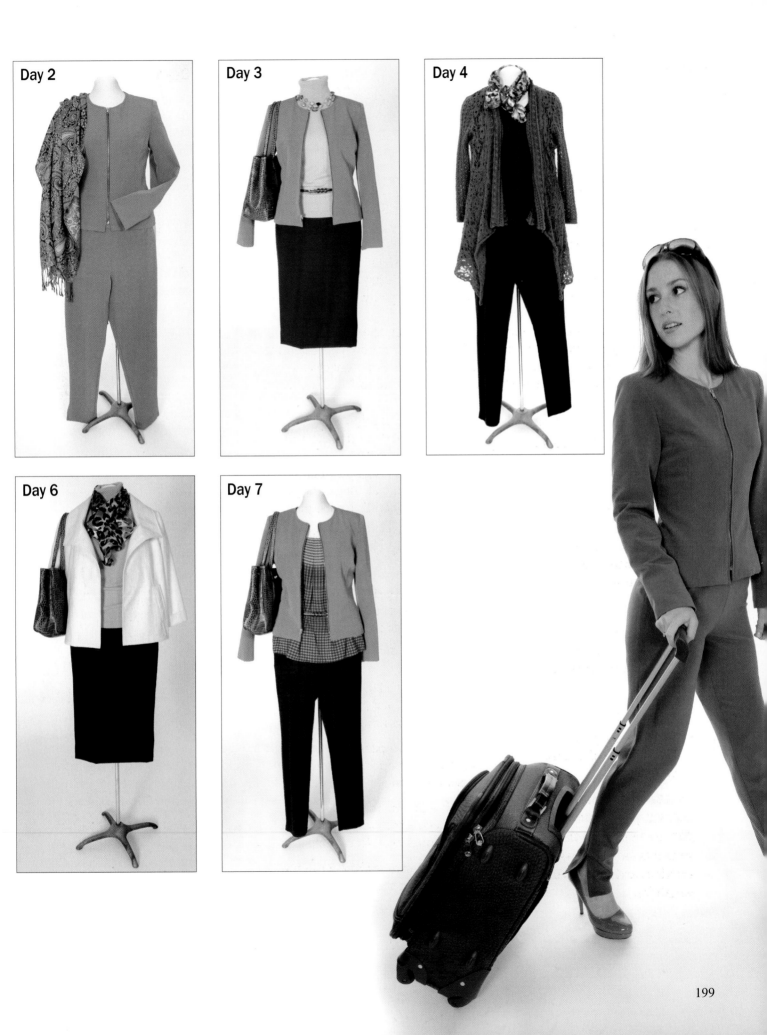

Day 2

Day 3

Day 4

Day 6

Day 7

199

It Pays to Plan

- Make a list of anticipated activities and what you'll need for each.

- A few days before your departure, pull the items you intend to take.

- Plan to get multiple uses for each garment you're packing. Mix and match them to be sure you have options for all the activities you've listed.

- Travel with garments you've worn successfully before; this is no time for surprises.

Plan Major Pieces First

- Use neutral colors for your main pieces so everything goes with everything. Darker neutrals and prints camouflage minor soil and wrinkles.

- Pack easy-care fabrics like washable, drip-dry synthetics. New manmade fibers wick moisture away from your body so they are cool and comfortable even for adventure travel. Knits wrinkle far less than most woven fabrics. Soft fabrics often wrinkle less than crisp ones.

- Most tops should go with most bottoms. Extra tops are lightweight to pack and extend your coordination options.

- Include a lightweight dark pant that can go from day into evening. Your best neutral should coordinate with nearly every top in your wardrobe. Add a glitzy wrap and earrings and you're ready for a night on the town.

- Pack items that can do double duty, like a shirt that can double as a lightweight jacket.

- Expect temperature extremes and pack layers you can add or subtract accordingly.

- Choose your coat for the climate but always be prepared for rain. A lightweight nylon raincoat can be rolled into a tiny corner of your suitcase, and umbrellas can collapse to just inches.

Security Tip

To protect against pickpockets or thieves, consider wearing a shoulder bag with the strap over your head and across your body. Be sure the strap is adjusted so the bag hangs at the top of your hip bone and in front of your body, where you can watch it. This keeps your hands free, your valuables safe, and is much more stylish than a hip pack.

The Necessary Extras

- Accessories change the look of basic pieces. Use color accents in scarves and jewelry to spice up your solid-color garments.

- Don't risk losing your fine jewelry. Take only the pieces you wear every day.

- Shoes are heavy, but by planning your clothes in a unified color palette, you can probably limit yourself to one casual pair and one dressier pair. Substitute comfy socks for bedroom slippers.

- Take one handbag that works with everything, and pack a flat clutch for evening if necessary. Consider a lightweight foldaway tote for sightseeing and souvenir shopping.

- Airplanes can be chilly, so tuck a cozy pashmina shawl and pair of socks into your carry-on bag.

- Get quadruple mileage from a lightweight knit pant and pullover. It's casual wear around the hotel, a workout uniform, swim cover-up and even sleepwear … all in just two pieces.

Packing Pointers

Suitcase Selection

- Choose lightweight luggage with reinforced corners, built-in wheels, and a pull-out handle. Some travelers prefer backpacks, many of which come with highly organized internal compartments and zip on/zip off external components as well.

- A carry-on bag may be all you need if you've planned your travel capsule carefully. But a larger suitcase lets you lay jackets, skirts and blouses flat with few, if any, folds. That means fewer wrinkles when you arrive—a bargain if your airline offers complimentary luggage checking.

A structured hanging garment bag—one that folds in half to carry—is another good choice. Drape pants or a skirt over the bar of a hanger, and add a blouse and jacket for most efficient use of space. Fold a dress over the bar of a separate hanger, and pin or clip at the waist.

Remove all previous routing tags before checking your luggage. And double-check the new tags to be sure your bags are headed to the same destination you are.

ALWAYS have name tags both inside and outside your bags.

Mark nondescript bags with distinctive colorful tags or decorative tape so you can recognize them easily on the carousel and nobody else will mistake them for theirs.

Pack Like a Pro

Always pack well ahead of departure time and make a complete checklist. Take the list along in your carry-on in case your bags are lost. And use it to be sure you pack everything for the return trip.

Pack valuables, medication and clean undies in your carry-on … just in case.

Pack heavy items like shoes at the bottom end of the suitcase, by the wheels. Non-crushable items like sweaters and lingerie go next, with more easily wrinkled items on top.

Consider packing garments on their own hangers and in plastic dry-cleaner bags to minimize wrinkling. The bags retain enough air to cushion the garment, and the hangers make unpacking a breeze. This is one time it's okay to use the thin metal hangers from the cleaners instead of heavier tubular or swivel-head styles.

To pack pants, leave the extra leg length hanging over the edge of the suitcase while you pack other clothes on top. Then fold the legs over the other layers to avoid a defined fold that can form a crease. Handle dresses the same way.

Alternate the direction of necklines and bottoms as you pack blouses and jackets.

Pack a thin robe and your slipper/socks on top so you can get to them first and finish unpacking in cozy comfort.

Travel Tips & Tidbits

Clear zip-top bags are travel lifesavers. Pack undies in one, scarves in one, nylons in one and so on. Carry extras to use along the way for damp swimsuits and dirty laundry.

To prevent soiling clothes, pack each shoe in an individual cloth or plastic bag. (Individual bags tuck into smaller areas better than bags made to hold a pair.)

Keep shoes in shape by stuffing the toes with tissue paper, or with small items like socks.

Place firm leather belts around the perimeter of the suitcase. Roll softer ones and tuck into corners or shoes.

Pack travel sizes of toiletries. You can make your own by refilling the bottles from complimentary hotel items with your favorite brands from home.

Of course you'll put all the liquids in a separate zip-top bag for security screening if you plan to carry your bag on an airplane.

Take your share of free perfume samples from the cosmetic counter. The tiny vials are perfect for travel.

Use a picnic salt shaker with a snap-on lid for your favorite bath powder. Try an empty prescription bottle for face powder; choose one that's the right size for your powder brush.

A small roll of masking tape can double as a lint remover. Just wrap a length of tape around your hand, sticky side out. And use it to seal cosmetic bottles to prevent leaks. In a pinch it can even work to hold up a loose hem.

A week's worth of great outfits in a carry-on bag.

- Moist towelettes in individual foil packets are great portable stain removers, even for makeup.

- Keep a mini sewing kit in your suitcase. You can make your own with a needle, a few safety and straight pins, and a few basic thread colors wrapped around a bit of cardboard. Stash it all in a used prescription bottle. You can include a small scissors unless you're wanting to carry the sewing kit onto an airplane; even the tiniest pair won't make it through security.

- Assemble a mini first aid kit in a metal Band-Aid box, including whatever remedies you consistently use at home.

- Slip the barrel of your curling iron into a cardboard tube to protect your clothing if you must pack it while it's still hot.

- Keep necklace chains from tangling by cutting a drinking straw to half the length of the chain, sliding one end through the straw and then securing the clasp.

When You Arrive

Give your clothes a steam bath. If you've used plastic drycleaner bags, remove them and store them in your suitcase so the housekeeping staff doesn't throw them away. Hang the garments from the shower curtain rod, away from the water source.

Turn on the hot water (be sure the drain is open) to build up steam. Close the door tightly and in as little as 10 minutes everything will look freshly pressed. Then allow the steam to humidify your entire hotel room.

For Frequent Flyers

It's worth the investment to keep a set of travel necessities always packed so you're ready at a moment's notice. Adapt this list to your personal needs:

- Duplicate cosmetics and toiletries.

- Manicure set including individual packets of polish remover.

- Shower cap and disposable razors.

- Travel-sized hair appliances—dryer, flat iron, and so on.

- Travel iron or steamer.

- Extension cord—hotel outlets never seem to be where you need them.

- Phone and computer charging devices.

- Adapters and voltage converters needed in foreign countries.

- Heating pad for achy muscles and cold rooms.

- Spot remover.

- Lightweight nightie and robe.

- Swimsuit, workout wear.

- Collapsible umbrella and hat, sunglasses.

- Favorite coffees, tea bags, hot chocolate, dry soup mix, oatmeal.

- Mini stapler, tape, paper clips.

- Letterhead, envelopes, post cards, stamps.

- Ear plugs to keep out hotel noise.

For more detailed travel and packing tips, check out Smart Packing For Today's Traveler by Susan Foster. See smartpacking.com for more family packing and airport security tips and to sign up for her free newsletter. Also see Leslie Willmott's website, smartwomenonthego.com.

Index

Resources Available from Author Nancy Nix-Rice

For style inspiration, in-person and long-distance color consulting, wardrobe consultations, and booking inquiries for programs on style and wardrobe development, you can connect with author Nancy Nix-Rice:

- through NancyNixRice.com and LookingGoodBook.com
- via email at NNR@NancyNixRice.com
- by phone at 314-803-4445
- on facebook.com/nancy.nixrice
- at linkedin.com/in/nancynixrice
- on pinterest.com/nancynixrice/
- at instagram.com/LookingGoodOnTheStreet for photos of women illustrating points of connection

McCall Pattern Company Photos

Thanks to McCall Pattern Company for allowing the use of photos of its designs from the from the McCall's, Vogue, and Butterick pattern catalogs. If you like a design, find it by page number. Go to ccallpattern.com, search by pattern number, and order it. But remember, designs get discontinued. All patterns are subject to availability and are copyrighted by the McCall Pattern Company. Images below courtesy of the McCall Pattern Company copyright ©2013.

Resources

There are many fine products and services to support your wardrobe development. Below are some resources we have used and recommend. There are undoubtedly other good ones we have not personally sampled. Omitting an item does not imply that we regard it negatively.

Color Consultants

- Nancy Nix-Rice – St. Louis, Mo. in-person and long-distance consultations. *LookingGoodBook.com*
- Ethel Harms – Portland, Ore. *YourImageConsultant.com*
- Dominique Isbecque, AICI, CIP, Image Resource Center of New York *ircny.com*
- Elaine Stoltz – Fort Worth, Tex. *StoltzImage.com*
- Beryl Wing, AICI, CIP The Image Authority Staten Island, N.Y. *theimageauthority.com*

Custom Clothiers

- Association of Sewing and Design Professionals (ASDP) – A national organization providing advanced training and certification for highly skilled sewing professionals, with members in most major cities. *sewingprofessionals.org*

Image & Wardrobe

Many of the reviewers of this book, along with the author herself, do image and wardrobe consulting. Please look for them online for more information.

Hidden Accessories

- Shoulder Shapes – removable foam pads with natural shaping and an unglazed finish to cling to garment fabric. *LookingGoodBook.com*
- Sleeve Bands – expandable metal "garters" to keep sleeves pushed up. *LookingGoodBook.com*
- Invisibelt – flat, undetectable and adjustable belt keeps waistbands snug and closures flat. *Invisibelt.com*
- Toeless pantyhose – great for open-toed shoes. *Silkies.com, Hanes.com* or *Hue.com*

There are countless sources for fashions and accessories. In addition to traditional retail stores, we enjoy supporting entrepreneurial women and the companies that supply them, such as:

Fashion Jewelry

- Premier Designs. *Premierdesigns.com*
- Stella & Dot. *Stelladot.com*
- Silpada. *Silpada.com*
- Nancy's personal picks for color links. *LookingGoodBook.com*

Handbags

- Miche – base handbag shapes with interchangeable magnetic covers. *Miche.com*
- Beijo – high-gloss pearlized bags in rainbow colors. *Beijobags.com*

Scarves

- Nancy's personal picks for color links. Includes videos demonstrating scarf tying. *LookingGoodBook.com*

Clothing

- CAbi – Affordable designer coordinates available through in-home trunk shows. *CAbionline.com*
- Carlisle/PerSe – Upscale separates, extensively coordinated, sold through independent consultants. *CarlisleCollection.com*
- Doncaster – Upscale coordinates and dresses, sold through independent consultants. *Doncaster.com*

Undergarments

- Jockey – new Volumetric fitting system lets you test cup sizes and custom-order the ideal band and cup combination for your figure. Company-owned stores and online ordering. *Jockey.com*
- Wacoal – high quality, beautiful bras and panties, available through better department stores. Company experts offer in-store fitting events, sometimes with donations to breast cancer research. *Wacoal-america.com*
- Soma Intimates – lingerie specialty store featuring lovely bras in an extensive size range. Many incorporate "vanishing back" design. Locations in malls nationwide. *Soma.com*

- Spanx – shaper undergarments to smooth and slim your body. And check out their affordable Assets collection too. *Spanx.com*
- NoNonsense – affordable fashion and shaping legwear. Check out Great Shapes and Shoe Solutions. Discounts through their online hosiery club. *NoNonsense.com*

Wardrobe Organizing Apps

- For Apple devices: Stylebook is the app featured in this book (page 162). Other options include Cloth, Closet+ and I wear.
- For Android devices: Options include ClosetVirtual, Personal Closet, and MyCloset

For readers who are also sewing enthusiasts...

Fashion Fabrics & Patterns

If you are fortunate to have an independent fashion fabric retailer in your area, by all means support them with your business. And seek out and patronize similar stores when you travel.

- Sawyer Brook – a fine online fabric retailer specializing in color-coordinated collections that are ideal for creating capsule wardrobes like those shown in Chapter 11. *SawyerBrook.com*
- Search the Internet for other fabric retailers doing online business such as Vogue Fabrics, Evanston, Ill., *voguefabricsstore.com*, and Fabric Depot, Portland, Ore., *fabricdepot.com*
- Fashion Patterns: *mccall.com, butterick.mccall.com, voguepattern.mccall.com, simplicity.com* Palmer/Pletsch patterns for McCall's provide fitting help. Search online for additional pattern companies.

Palmer/Pletsch, the publisher of this book, is known as "The Fashion Sewing Authority" and Pati Palmer is McCall's Fit Expert. The next three pages list Palmer/Pletsch books and DVDs, including those relevant to image: *Looking Good—Live DVD*, *Full Busted? Sew Clothes That Fit DVD*, two fit DVDs, and books on fitting and pant fitting and sewing.

LOOK FOR THESE PRODUCTS FROM PALMER/PLETSCH:

Books on Fit, Fashion & Fabric

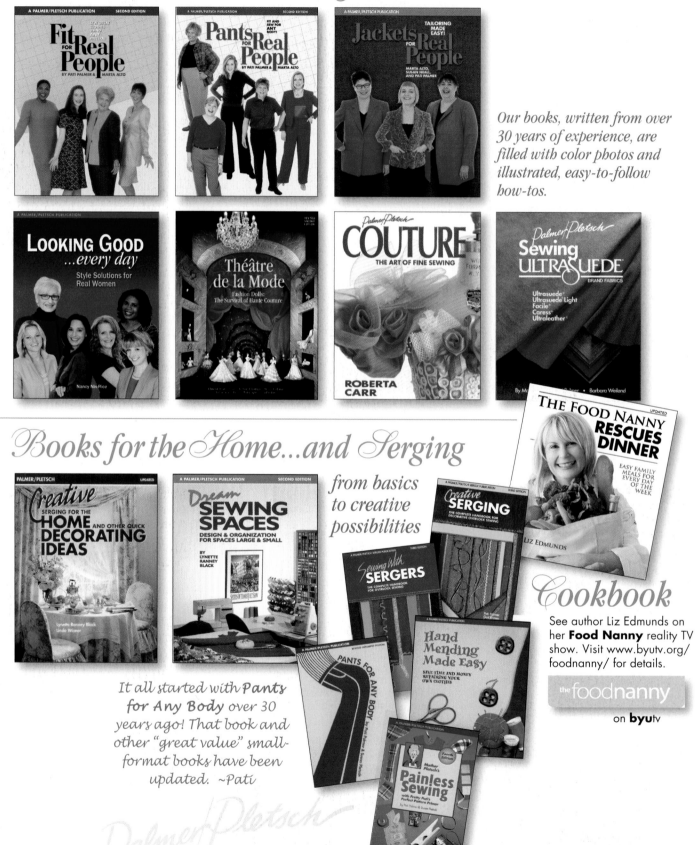

Our books, written from over 30 years of experience, are filled with color photos and illustrated, easy-to-follow how-tos.

Books for the Home...and Serging

from basics to creative possibilities

Cookbook

See author Liz Edmunds on her **Food Nanny** reality TV show. Visit www.byutv.org/foodnanny/ for details.

the foodnanny
on **byu**tv

It all started with **Pants for Any Body** over 30 years ago! That book and other "great value" small-format books have been updated. ~Pati

INTERACTIVE
DVDs

The styles and techniques in our books are brought to life and expanded on by Marta Alto and Pati Palmer in these DVD videos.

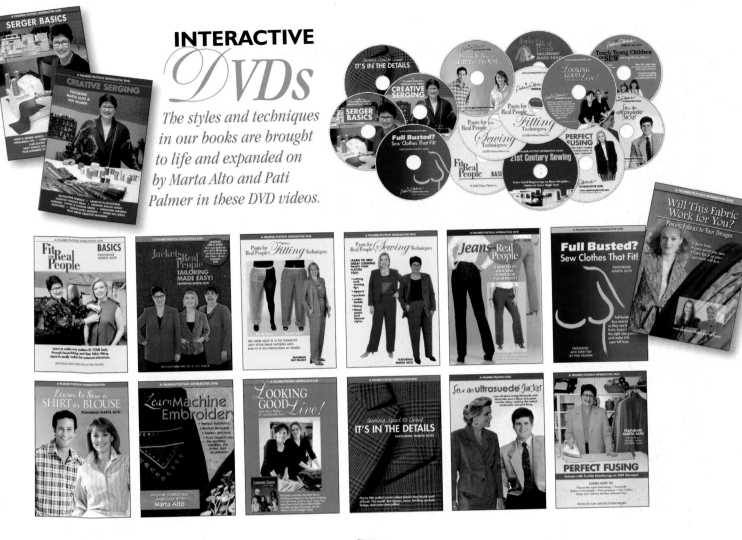

Children Love to Sew...

My First Sewing Books and Kits,
by Winky Cherry Along with a teaching manual and DVD, they offer a complete, thoroughly tested sewing program for children ages 5 to 11.

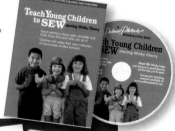

Patterns

Palmer/Pletsch for McCall's are the McCall Pattern Company's top-selling patterns.

Also look for our *Learn to Sew!* **Teacher-in-an-Envelope**

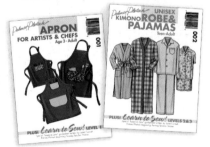

And don't miss the FREE

FASHION FOR
Real PEOPLE
ONLINE MAGAZINE

User-Friendly Interfacings

PerfectFuse™

- ◆ Developed BY sewers FOR sewers.
- ◆ These four distinctly different products cover 90% of interfacing needs.
- ◆ Come in convenient 1-yard and 3-yard packages
- ◆ Extra wide for cutting larger pattern pieces
- ◆ Each interfacing has its own separate use, care and how-to instructions.
- ◆ All four weights available in charcoal-black and ecru-white

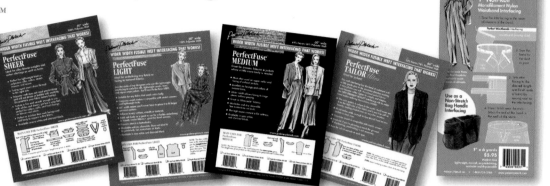

PERFECT SEW NEEDLE THREADER

Now thread both machine and hand needles with ease. On one end of this tool is the specially designed hook that makes threading easy. The other end is an integrated needle inserter for both conventional and serger machine needles.

threading hand needles

threading machine needles

inserting machine needles

PERFECT PATTERN PAPER
two 84" x 48" sheets

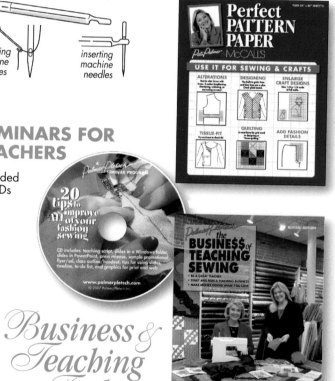

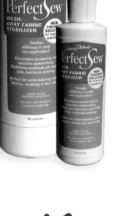

SEMINARS FOR TEACHERS

provided on CDs

Business & Teaching Tools

PALMER/PLETSCH *Workshops* *Take A Sewing Vacation!*

Our "Sewing Vacations" are offered on a variety of sewing and fit topics. Workshops are held at the Palmer/Pletsch Training Center in Portland, Oregon, and at satellite locations around the country.

Teacher training sessions available on some topics include practice teaching sessions, digital slides and teaching script; camera-ready workbook handouts, and publicity flyer.

Visit www.palmerplesch.com for a complete schedule.

For more details on these and other products, workshops, and teacher training, please visit our website:

www.palmerpletsch.com

Palmer/Pletsch Publishing
1801 N.W. Upshur Street, Suite 100, Portland, OR 97209
(503) 274-0687 or fax (503) 274-1377
or 1-800-728-3784 (orders)
info@palmerpletsch.com